COUPLE CONNECTION MASTERY

THE HIGH-PERFORMANCE RELATIONSHIP FRAMEWORK FOR ENGINEERING UNBREAKABLE LOVE IN 28 DAYS: STRENGTHEN TRUST, DEEPEN INTIMACY AND IMPROVE COMMUNICATION

DARYL PARSONS

PARSONS PRESS

COPYRIGHT AND THERAPEUTIC DISCLAIMER

Copyright © 2025 by Daryl Parsons – MNZCCA - Licensed Professional Counselor

All rights reserved.

No part of this book may be reproduced, scanned, stored or transmitted in any printed or electronic form without permission. It is illegal to copy this book, post it to a website, or distribute it by any other means without permission. Please do not participate in or encourage piracy of copyrighted materials in violation of the author's rights. Thank you for respecting the hard work of this author.

Daryl Parsons asserts the moral right to be identified as the author of this work.

Daryl Parsons has no responsibility for the persistence or accuracy of URLs for external or third-party internet websites referred to in this publication and does not guarantee that any content on such websites is, or will remain, accurate or appropriate.

Designations used by companies to distinguish their products are often claimed as trademarks. All brand names and product names used in this book and on its cover are trade names, service marks, trademarks and registered trademarks of their respective owners. The publishers and the book are not associated with any product or vendor mentioned in this book. None of the companies named in this book have endorsed it.

Therapeutic Disclaimer:

All couple stories included herein are based on real characters but have been merged and altered to ensure client stories are unidentifiable. Any perceived likeness between the characters referred to and actual individuals is purely coincidental. The author has no responsibility or legal liability for how the guidance and contents in this book are applied toward improving personal relationships or wellbeing.

While the author provides psychological services, this book is not a substitute for couple therapy, diagnosis or treatment of medical or psychological problems. If you require medical, psychological, or other expert assistance, consult your physician or licensed professional counselor.

SEVEN REASONS WHY YOU CAN TRUST ME AS YOUR COACH:

A - I have invested 35 years in helping young people, working for 20 of those years (from 2005-2025) as a therapist and educator, including clinically supervising counselling degree students during their practicum years through to graduation and beyond.

B - I am experienced in trauma and couple therapy; clinical leadership; business sales and management; counsellor education; leadership coaching; men's research; crisis response leadership; mental health, emotional wellbeing and suicide prevention workshops for leaders. I love growing whole people, strong couples and families, holistic businesses and organizations, for a more loving healthy society and eternal impact.

C - I earned a Master of Counselling with Merit from the University of Canterbury.

D - I am committed to personally growing as I receive regular clinical supervision and counselling. This has included receiving couple and family counselling. I am an avid reader and participant in learning from courses, coaching, conferences and training events. There are no untested theories here. It is all lived, real, proven and effective.

4 | SEVEN REASONS WHY YOU CAN TRUST ME AS YOUR COACH:

E - Delightful Tomomi and I have been married since November 2020, as we've re-built our family life between New Zealand and Japan. I learnt much while married to Melissa from 2002-2018, when she sadly died of cancer. In the last six years I have grown through widowhood, grief and single parenting – into new, stronger, deeper love – thanks to my empathic God, wife and support people. Now I write for and coach others in these areas.

F - Clinically, I utilize aspects of Person-Centred Therapy, Narrative, Imago, Existential, Solution Focused, CBT, Somatic and Internal Family Systems Therapies, amongst others. I am clinically licensed to use the Prepare-Enrich couple assessments and materials.

G - I work with couples who are stuck in disconnection patterns, conflict, pornography, mental illness, habits and addictions, intergenerational trauma, suicidality and abuse - to rebuild safe attachment and emotional attunement, as they reconstruct their lives and relationships. See my Therapeutic Disclaimer on the Copyright page.

NOTE: This book is specifically for those who find themselves disconnected and conflicted. It is NOT designed for the other situations listed above, which need more intensive care, therapy and group courses to heal and grow in sustainable ways.

To view a brief explanatory video from Daryl, scan the QR Code below.

King Solomon experienced and wrote this about love 3000 years ago:

> [7] Again I saw something meaningless under the sun:
> [8] There was a man all alone; he had neither son nor brother. There was no end to his toil, yet his eyes were not content with his wealth. "For whom am I toiling," he asked, "and why am I depriving myself of enjoyment?"
> This too is meaningless – a miserable business!
> [9] Two are better than one, because they have a good return for their labor: [10] If either of them falls down, one can help the other up. But pity anyone who falls and has no one to help them up. [11] Also, if two lie down together, they will keep warm. But how can one keep warm alone? [12] Though one may be overpowered, two can defend themselves. A cord of three strands is not quickly broken.
>
> — KING SOLOMON, ECCLESIASTES 4:7-11 (NIV)

His cherished spouse exclaimed: *"I have found the one whom my soul loves."*

— SONG OF SOLOMON 3:4 (NIV)

With all my heart felt love and appreciation...
To my wife Tomomi Nabeshima-Parsons, who loved me back to life through widowhood, grief and single-parenting - into thriving and prospering.
Thank you for bringing so much empathy,

sparkle,

positivity,

fun,

laughter,

travel,

family,

learning,

beauty,

and joy into my life.
Bi-culturally and bi-lingually!
Without your committed friendship and love, I would not be flourishing like this..
Nor could I write this book to help couples grow unbreakable love like we have.
Arigato guzaimasu. Tomo wa watashi no Yorokobi! Zuto Aishiteru.
You're the best thing that's ever happened to me - Tomomi!

CONTENTS

Introduction	13

Part I
DECODE

1. THE PARTNERSHIP DRIFT	33
Recognizing the Subtle Signs of Emotional Drift	35
Understanding the Logistics-Only Trap	36
Breaking the Cycle: With 6-Minute Love Habits	39
The Science Behind the Shift	41
Breaking the Cycle of Postponed Connection	43
Closing Reflection - Success Story	44
2. TIME-STARVED LOVE	47
Debunking the Quality Time Myth	49
The Power of Micro-Moments for Engineering Connection	52
The Science of Micro-Connection	53
Strategic Connection in a Busy World	55
Closing Reflection	58
3. THE SCIENCE OF CONNECTION	59
Understanding Emotional Bandwidth	61
Measuring Relationship Vitality	62
RELATIONSHIP VITALITY DASHBOARD FOR COUPLE CONNECTION MASTERY	67
Closing Reflection	71
4. ENGINEERING LOVE	73
Introducing the Couple Connection Engineering System	75
Your 28-Day Transformation Roadmap to Better Connection:	77
Closing Reflection - Success Story	79

Part II
ENGINEER

5. THE RELATIONSHIP BUILD FRAMEWORK - YOUR BLUEPRINT FOR SUCCESS — 83
   - Explaining the Five Phases of B.U.I.L.D for Engineering Unbreakable Love — 85
   - Setting Measurable Outcomes and Implementation Strategies — 87
   - The Power of Love Habits in Connecting with Nature — 89
   - Closing Reflection and Success Story — 89

6. BASE - FOUNDATION SETTING — 91
   - Assessment Tools and Metrics — 94
   - Goal Alignment Strategies — 95
   - Couple Connection Methods - The Technology of Touch — 96
   - Closing Reflection and Success Story: Recording Your Couple Connection Quality Across Your 28-Day Roadmap — 96

7. UNDERSTAND - CONNECTION MAPPING — 101
   - Daily Interaction Analysis - Understanding Connection Mapping — 103
   - Trigger Identification — 105
   - Couple Stories and Closing Reflections — 107

8. IMPLEMENT - STRATEGIC CONNECTION POINTS — 109
   - Morning Ritual Design — 111
   - Midday Check-in Optimization — 113
   - Evening Bonding Habits — 114
   - Closing Reflection and Success Story — 116

9. LEVERAGE - SYSTEM OPTIMIZATION — 119
   - Pattern Refinement — 121
   - Success Amplification — 122
   - Strategy Scaling — 123
   - Couple Stories Illustrating Leverage — 124
   - Closing Reflection and Success Story — 125

10. DEEPEN - ARCHITECTURE STRENGTHENING — 127
    - Practice Integration — 129
    - Routine Establishment — 130
    - System Maintenance — 131
    - Closing Reflection and Success Story — 133

Part III
FORTIFY

11. **CRISIS-PROOFING YOUR CONNECTION** — 139
    - Why Crisis-Proofing Your Connection Matters — 141
    - Designing Your Emergency Response Protocols — 142
    - Rapid Reconnection Techniques — 143
    - Stress-Tested Bonding Strategies — 144
    - Success Story: The Pandemic Pivot — 145

12. **LONG-DISTANCE ENGINEERING** — 149
    - The Value of Long-Distance Engineered Love — 151
    - Virtual Connection Design — 151
    - Remote Intimacy Building — 153
    - Digital Bonding Protocols — 153
    - Closing Reflection — 156

13. **CAREER-CONNECTION INTEGRATION** — 157
    - Professional Boundary Setting — 159
    - Work-Home Synergy Creation — 160
    - Winning with Achievement and Intimacy — 161
    - Success Stories: How Two Couples Tracked their Progress — 163
    - Closing Reflection — 164

14. **FAMILY SYSTEM INTEGRATION** — 167
    - Parenting Partnership Alignment — 169
    - Extended Family Navigation — 170
    - United Front Engineering — 172
    - Measuring Family Connection and Repair Processes in Four of Our Global Families — 173
    - Their tracking system was an elegantly simple poster on the pantry: — 174
    - Closing Reflection — 176

15. **SOCIAL CONNECTION ARCHITECTURE** — 177
    - Couple Identity Development — 179
    - Community Integration Strategies — 180
    - Support Network Building — 181
    - Couple Identity in Community - Noticing Progress with Three of Our Couples — 183
    - Closing Reflection — 184

16. ADVANCED CONNECTION ENGINEERING	187
Next-Level Intimacy Techniques	189
Innovation in Connection Practices	190
Imagining Your Preferred Future	191
Advanced Connection Engineering - Celebrating Mastery with Two of our Couples	192
Closing Reflection	194

CONCLUSION

17. YOUR ENGINEERING LEGACY	199
Valuing Your Engineering Legacy as a Treasure to Share	200
Maintaining Momentum	202
Creating Lasting Impact	204
What You Do Locally Can Help Couple Connection Improve Globally	205
APPENDICES	209
References	217
Also Written by Daryl Parsons	223

INTRODUCTION

THE INTIMACY-ACHIEVEMENT PARADOX

Your system is perfectly designed to be giving you the results you are currently getting

— W. EDWARDS DEMMING

Real Life Scenario: Business Success vs Crumbling Marriage

Sarah stared at her CEO of the Year award, ruing why such remarkable success felt so hollow.

Her tech company had just topped $100 million in revenue, yet her marriage was silently crumbling. That morning, her husband Michael, a managing partner at a consulting firm, had left another breakfast untouched – their eighth consecutive day without a real conversation.

Both had tried everything: scheduling date nights (interrupted by urgent calls), couples therapy (missed sessions due to board meetings), and weekend getaways (spent checking emails). Their professional skills that built empires now seemed powerless to rebuild their connection.

The breakthrough came in a product development meeting. As Sarah reviewed her team's system architecture diagram, she recognized a familiar pattern. "*We map user touchpoints, measure engagement, and optimize interactions,*" she thought. "*Why aren't we applying these same principles at home?*"

That night, she shared her insight with Michael. His eyes lit up - *finally, an approach that spoke their language.* Together, they began treating their relationship like their most important project, applying the same analytical rigor that made them successful at work.

Disconnected High-Performance Couples Often Ask Questions Like:

- How did we go from being in love to feeling like business partners?
- Is it possible to rebuild intimacy with our hectic schedules?
- Are we too far gone, or is there still hope for us to reconnect?
- How can we fix our relationship without sacrificing our careers?

THE HIDDEN COST OF CAREER SUCCESS ON RELATIONSHIPS

Like Sarah and Michael, 72% of high-achieving professionals report decreased relationship satisfaction during career growth phases. This isn't due to lack of commitment - it's a systems problem waiting for an engineering solution.

Professional Success Metrics vs. Relationship Impact

Career Achievement	Relationship Challenge	Hidden Cost
Revenue growth	Decreased quality time	68% Report missing key moments
Project success	Reduced communication	74% Cite work interruptions
Market leadership	Emotional distance	65% Feel disconnected

This pattern emerges not from lack of care or commitment, but from misapplied professional strengths. Your analytical abilities and process optimization skills aren't the problem - they're actually the solution.

As the father of systems improvement, W. Edwards Demming said, *"your system is designed to give you the results you are currently getting."* His observation holds an invitation to assess your results first, in order to learn how to improve your system.

Why Busy Professionals Need Realistic and Systematic Relationship Advice

Some relationship advice can feel removed from your reality. *"Just spend more time together"* or *"communicate better"* lack the precision and measurability you've mastered in your work.

COMMON ADVICE VS. PROFESSIONAL REALITY

Traditional Approach: Schedule whole weekends for connection	**Reality:** Changeable work demands make this untenable	**Solution:** *Engineer micro-moments to fit your timetable*
Standard Guidance: Express feelings more openly	**Reality:** Analytical thinkers need structured frameworks	**Solution:** *Create measurable emotional connection habits*
Typical Recommendation: Prioritize relationship over work	**Reality:** Both are essential for fulfilment and wellbeing in life	**Solution:** *Design systems to optimize both concurrently*

Top performers know that identifying system behavior precedes optimization. Professional success comes by recognizing patterns, analyzing data and implementing systematic solutions.

Now it's time to apply these same skills to strengthen your relationship. The systematic approach driving your career achievements will be your template for relationship excellence. Your analytical mind isn't the problem - it's the solution you haven't fully leveraged yet.

When Sarah and Michael first walked into my office, the tension between them was palpable. As successful professionals in their early forties, they had achieved remarkable career feats but found their relationship crumbling under endless responsibilities and fading connection. Like many high-achieving couples, they juggled the demands of parenting, maintaining their health, caring for aging parents, and nurturing their social lives, all while striving to keep their love alive.

Over the course of 28 days, Sarah and Michael embarked on a transformative journey guided by the principles of *Couple Connection Mastery*. By integrating cutting-edge research, practical exercises, and a systematic approach tailored to their unique needs, they rebuilt their relationship from the ground up. They learned to decode the patterns that had led to their disconnection, engineer new love-habits that built trust and intimacy, and fortify their bond against future challenges.

This book introduces you to my powerful *Couple Connection Mastery* relationship framework, a high-performance system designed for analytically-minded couples like Sarah and Michael. It combines the precision of engineering with the wisdom of emotional intelligence to help you align your relationship success with your professional achievements. It does this aware that 'it takes a village to raise a couple,' with reliance on family, friends, workmates and supporters. Acknowledging that couple and family relationships deeply impact wider societal wellbeing.

Through a three-part framework - DECODE, ENGINEER, FORTIFY - you will learn to recognize the factors contributing to your current situation, implement practical strategies to strengthen your connection, and develop the skills to sustain your love in the face of life's demands. Each part builds upon the previous, guiding you from awareness to mastery, empowering you to create the relationship you've always envisioned.

What sets this ground-breaking approach apart is its focus on the unique challenges faced by high-achieving couples in the modern world. By blending evidence-based strategies with practical exercises designed for busy professionals, *Couple Connection Mastery* equips you with the tools to build an unbreakable bond in just 6 minutes a day, over 28 days.

As a licensed professional counselor, educator and former carpenter, I have 35 years of experience building strong foundations in structures and relationships. My 20 years of work in trauma therapy, couple counseling, business and leadership coaching has taught me that the key to a thriving relationship is in the daily habits and practices that shape our connections.

Through the pages of this book, you will discover how to strengthen trust, deepen intimacy, and improve communication, amidst the pressures of life. You will learn to navigate the challenges of long-distance relationships, integrate your career aspirations with your partnership, and orchestrate a harmonious family system that supports your growth.

By committing to this *Couple Connection Mastery* pathway, you can expect to experience a renewal of your relationship. You will develop a deeper understanding of yourselves and acquire habits to bond efficiently, forging robust emotional connection that will stand the test of time.

I invite you to seize the restorative potential of this book and commit to building unbreakable love. *Believe me – it is worth everything you put into it.* Together, we will decode the details of your current connection, engineer your relationship to thrive, and fortify your bond against life's challenges. Let's travel the road toward *Couple Connection Mastery*, one loving habit at a time.

CHECKING COUPLE CONNECTION WITHIN A WHOLE OF SYSTEM LIFE QUALITY OVERVIEW

To understand where your couple relationship sits in the bigger picture and how this affects it, I invite you to assess the quality of your lives before we take further steps together. *Why?* For the same reason you don't just check the spark plugs without assessing the overall engine function in your car. You need to know how your relationship is impacted by, and affects, the rest of your life, to keep the greater context in mind while working on your couple connection.

I have noticed in two decades of therapeutic and educational work with individuals, couples, families, workplaces, and organizations, how life is a dynamic interplay of many parts. These all contribute to the holistic wellbeing of people and societies. This universal human goal is known as success, prosperity, flourishing, quality of life, or similar - in various places and languages.

Checking Your Concept of Success or Richness of Life – What Your Target Looks Like

The value of pausing to think on these things must be recognized. Are we human beings or human doings? It is worth stepping back from our busy 'hamster wheel' of doing life's daily tasks to check why we are doing them and what sort of people we are being in the process.

It can be empowering to ask ourselves questions, such as, *"What does success mean to me? And why?"* And *"What does richness of life really look like?"*

For example, do we want to be *connection rich* in our relationships, families, friendships, workplaces, recreational, cultural, and spiritual activities and to enrich our communities? Or have we adopted a shallow, monodimensional story like, *"being rich only refers to having money or assets?"* A wider concept of wealth or flourishing across the system or 10 Dimensions below is more meaningful, as *"the sum of the whole is greater than that of the individual parts."*

International longitudinal research studies like The Blue Zones project show that people who build their lives on a collectivist holistic wellbeing model for the good of their communities tend to develop richer interpersonal relationships, vocational purpose, business achievement, and mental-emotional health. This combines with ecological harmony and fruitfulness, spiritual and cultural identity, as well as strong physical and recreational health. The results suggest that true wealth that enriches everyone is an achievable sociological enterprise, worthy of our attention.

Therefore, it will pay to consider what narrative is 'storying us' - as the story at the heart of our lives will show our ultimate values and how we use our power to embody those. For example, our use of our time, voice, energy, and money tells us what we value. *But how do we check this?*

The *'Whole of System – Time Use and Life Quality'* exercise below invites you to look at this via the societal context of your life, in which your individual, couple, family, and workplace well-being happens. *Think about how your couple relationship is formed by and influences your community.*

Remember, the analogy - we are 'checking the spark plugs' - of your couple connection, in light of the overall 'quality of function of your engine and vehicle' - the rest of your life. In this 20-minute exercise, record how you spend your time and energy in an average day and week. Let me first explain the function and purpose of the *'Whole of System – Time Use and Life Quality'* Chart, so you understand it. There are 10 evident dimensions to being an adult, which are listed in the left column of the Chart as *'Wellbeing Aspects'*. The next column called *'Human Behaviours'* simply lists the sorts of things we do behaviourally in each of those areas of daily life. The third column called *'Daily Being-Doing'* is where you take a brief snapshot - like a time and motion study - *of what you actually spend your time doing each day and how well it is working for you.*

Michael and Sarah's lived reality is recorded in the example Chart, showing you what their 24-hour days typically looked like, and how that mapped across to their 168-hour weekly time use.

Note that the *Daily* hours x7 does not neatly compute into the *Weekly* hours spent in each area, because more time was spent on those aspects on their weekends. For example, *'Physical and Bodily Health'* actions took 9 hours Daily, which could mean x7 = 63 hours Weekly, but Sarah and Michael spent longer making meals on weekends, so their Weekly total was 66 hours. For another example, they spent 2 hours Daily on *'Family'* activities, which could = 14 hours Weekly, but took an extra hour on the weekend, thus their Weekly total on *Familial* tasks was 15 hours.

Lastly, and most importantly – Michael and Sarah recorded spending 0.5 hours Daily together, which could mean x7 = 3.5 hours Weekly, but they spent more time as a couple on Sundays. This is why they wrote 5 for their total Weekly *'Relational'* Hours on the Chart.

And finally, the right-side column called *'Quality'* is their subjective rating of how well that aspect of being human is going for them right now, as a percentage score. They completed the 10 lines in the Chart and checked that their *Daily activities added up to 24 hours, then checked that their Weekly tasks added up to 168 hours*. To get their overall *Quality-of-Life Score*, they added up their felt *Quality* scores from the 10 lines and divided by 10 to get their average %.

On the bottom line of the Chart is the summary of their data from the whole exercise. It reads, *'Overall Quality of Life in 10 Dimensions with Total Time Use Daily / Weekly = 24 Hours = 168 Hours = 60%.'* Michael and Sarah measured the quality of their 10 *Wellbeing Aspects*, and after counting how each day and week was spent, their resulting *Quality-of-Life Score was 60%*. I hope this description and case study example helps this make sense and that you enjoy doing the exercise. It should be thought provoking – as it sets the scene for your couple connection.

Assess Couple Connection within Your Whole of System - Time Use and Life Quality

Worked example. Michael & Sarah's current Time Use, Wellbeing and Life Quality: (They did this separately then compared and averaged their hours on the chart)

Wellbeing Aspect	Human Behaviours	Daily Being-Doing	Daily	Weekly	Quality
Physical-Bodily	Bodily health actions	Sleep; food prep; eat-drink; wash; toilet;	9.0	66	65%
Mental-Emotional	Thinking-feeling-choosing	Nights Journalling	0.25	3	60%
Work-Study-Career	Vocation-calling-purpose	7am - 6pm x 5.5 days	11.0	64	75%
Familial-Generational	Family-relatives-support	Nights + Weekend	1.5	15	65%
Relational-Sexual	**Couplehood**-singlehood	**Nights + Weekend**	**0.5**	**5**	**40%**
Home-Assets-Financial	Property-bills-investments	Nights + Weekend	0.25	2	70%
Fun-Rest-Recreational	Exercise-hobbies-sports	Mornings + Weekend	0.5	5	55%
Spiritual-Cultural	Stories-values-practices	Nights Reflecting	0.25	2	50%
Social-Friends	Friend-community activities	In person + Online	0.5	4	65%
Natural-Ecological	Plants-animals-land-care	Nights + Weekend	0.25	2	55%
Overall Quality of Life in 10 Dimensions with Total Time Use Daily / Weekly:			**= 24 Hrs**	**=168 Hrs**	**60%**

Reflective Exercise:

We all have 86,400 seconds each day - what do you use yours for? Find out how much time you invest *Daily* and *Weekly* in your *10 Dimensions of Wellbeing* and what your felt *Quality-of-Life* is. This is as crucial as checking the function of your whole car engine, not just the spark plugs.

RECORD YOUR CURRENT TIME USE, WELLBEING AND LIFE QUALITY IN THIS CHART:

Wellbeing Aspect	Human Behaviours	Daily Being-Doing	Daily	Weekly	Quality
Physical-Bodily	Bodily health actions	Sleep; food prep; eat-drink; wash; toilet;			
Mental-Emotional	Thinking-feeling-choosing				
Work-Study-Career	Vocation-calling-purpose				
Familial-Generational	Family-relatives-support				
Relational-Sexual	Couplehood-singlehood				
Home-Assets-Financial	Property-bills-investments				
Fun-Rest-Recreational	Exercise-hobbies-sports				
Spiritual-Cultural	Stories-values-practices				
Social-Friends	Friend-community activities				
Natural-Ecological	Plants-animals-land-care				
Overall Quality of Life in 10 Dimensions with Total Time Use Daily / Weekly:			= 24 Hrs	=168 Hrs	

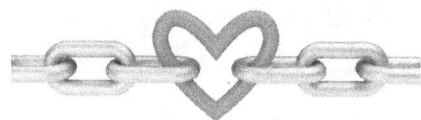

The Power of Couple Connection within Regular Whole of System Assessment

I expect this exercise was revealing for you, as it was for Sarah and Michael. They were shocked to find they only had 5 hours of connection time weekly and sad to rate their couple satisfaction at 40%. This is the power of combining quantitative and qualitative measurement together.

Now plot your Wellbeing Scores out of 10 for each dimension onto my *Holistic Individual and Societal Wellbeing Scale* below. Then join the dots of your plotted scores together to see the shape of your current wellbeing. To encourage you, this is not about failure or judgment, but about gaining a truthful, qualitative grasp of how your relationship fits within your whole life.

To illustrate, I have included Sarah and Michael's scores (with permission) from their *Whole of System Overview*, mapped onto the *Holistic Wellbeing Scale* below. They show the shape, the quality and quantity of their overall wellbeing at that time. This was before they responded to the

INTRODUCTION | 23

Final Reflection Task and enaged in *Couple Connection Mastery* to improve their couple connection, as is shown in the next chapter.

Michael and Sarah's Holistic Individual and Societal Wellbeing Scale

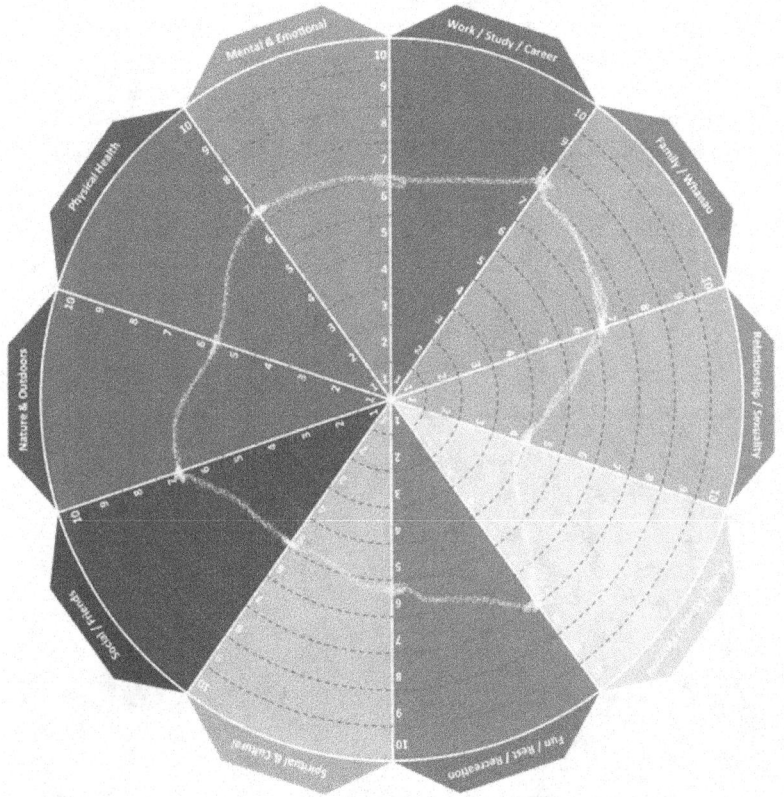

Final Reflection Task: Respond to the Wellbeing Scale questions below, to appreciate your current Wellbeing Score, and plan desired action steps with timeframes and strong support.

24 | INTRODUCTION

Appreciating and Strengthening Your Holistic Wellbeing – Towards Societal Wellbeing:

- How would you rate your Wellbeing in each related area, from 1 = Low, to 10 = High?
- Mark your scores on the Scale and join them up. What is your Wellbeing % Score? 60%
- Appreciate what you have achieved, with your support people. Well done, great work!
- Next, what area – if strengthened, would help your life the most? Couple Connection
- Brainstorm, how might you do this? Couple Connection Mastery and Daryl's Coaching
- Support – who could help you? Friends-Family And who could you help? Workmates
- When will you achieve this by? A months' time Who will notice? Us, kids, wider family
- Keep doing what works ☑ Check your progress often and update your support people

Now Complete Your Holistic Individual and Societal Wellbeing Scale

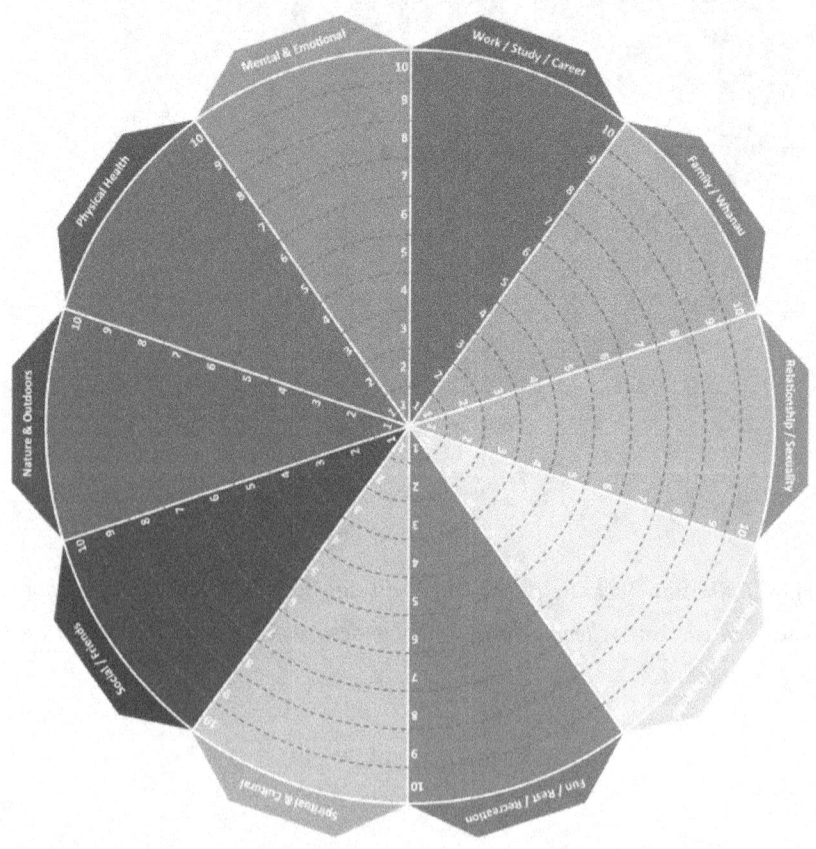

Final Reflection Task: Respond to the Wellbeing Scale questions below, to appreciate your current Wellbeing Score, and plan desired action steps with timeframes and strong support.

Appreciating and Strengthening Your Holistic Wellbeing – Towards Societal Wellbeing:

- How would you rate your Wellbeing in each related area, from 1 = Low, to 10 = High?
- Mark your scores on the Scale and join them up. What is your Wellbeing % Score?.....
- Appreciate what you have achieved, with your support people. Well done, great work!
- Next, what area – if strengthened, would help your life the most? ....
- Brainstorm, how might you do this? ....
- Support – who could help you? .... And who could you help? ....
- When will you achieve this by? .... Who will notice? ....
- Keep doing what works ☑ Check your progress often and update your support people

When entering your *Wellbeing* levels on the *Scale*, it can help to think of them as fluid, and to permit yourself to be in a mixture of survival, comfort and thriving states *all at the same time.* If that is the case, I get you! When I went through my former spouse Melissa's cancer journey with her in 2017-18, then her death and my subsequent widowhood, grief and single parenting journey with my boys, my *Wellbeing Score* was languishing between 40-50% for two years.

I shared my *Holistic Wellbeing Scale* with my Counsellor Dr Karey Meisner in 2018, and he saw I was self-scoring between 1-3 out of 10 in six dimensions. This can be seen as 'the red zone,' or *struggling for Survival*. He asked, *"how I was achieving this and not getting any worse?"* In three areas I scored between 4-6 out of 10, towards 'the orange zone,' or some *Comfort*. Surprisingly, in one area, I scored a 7/10, or 'green zone' towards *Thriving*. Giving myself permission to be in all three states at once was so validating and gave me so much more grace for myself. I truly appreciate Dr Karey for his empathic attention, astute insights and compassionate support.

Allowing for the *co-existence of survival, comfort and thriving in related areas of our lives at the same time is truthful and practical.* It can give us realistic expectations of ourselves, then help us tell our closest confidante how we really are and what they might do to best support us.

AN ENGINEERED APPROACH: YOUR WORK SUCCESS BLUEPRINT SHOWS THE COUPLE SOLUTION

Now you have a clear picture of your *Whole Life System*, let's work on your couple connection. As with professional excellence, relationship enhancement requires clear metrics, systematic analysis, and strategic optimization. Consider how you approach business challenges:

Professional Problem-Solving Pattern

1. Gather performance data
2. Analyze system behavior
3. Identify improvement opportunities
4. Design targeted solutions
5. Measure results
6. Optimize outcomes

This high-performance relationship framework transforms relationship improvement from guesswork into a precise science. *High achievers succeed by turning complex challenges into solvable equations - relationship patterns are no different.*

Sarah and Michael faced this challenge amid the flurry of innovation and ambition in their professions, embodying the quintessential modern dilemma. Both were titans in their fields, Sarah as CEO and Michael as a managing partner, and renowned for their ability to turn ideas into groundbreaking profitable technologies. Yet, within the realm of their relationship, they were at an impasse. Despite their professional triumphs, Sarah and Michael faced a chasm that seemed to widen with each passing day, threatening the very foundation of their union.

Their story typifies the task faced by many high-achieving couples who strive to excel both professionally and personally. I designed this book specifically for such couples, offering a high-performance relationship framework that promises to help you transform disconnection into a bond as agile and innovative as the careers you have forged.

THE ESSENCE OF COUPLE CONNECTION MASTERY

My strategic approach integrates engineering principles with emotional intelligence, recognizing that modern relationships require both analytical precision and heartfelt understanding. In crafting this book, I have drawn from my extensive background in counseling, business, and leadership coaching, along with my experiences in building structures and relationships.

The framework is structured in three distinct phases - DECODE, ENGINEER, and FORTIFY - that serve as the sequence for your relationship's metamorphosis. Each phase is explained below and is meticulously planned to build upon the last, guiding you through a process of noticing existing patterns, implementing new strategies, and securing the longevity of your connection.

THE 28-DAY TRANSFORMATIONAL ROADMAP – IN 3 PHASES

DECODE Phase (Days 1-7)

The DECODE Phase is the starting point of your relationship transformation. This initial stage is akin to examining the foundation of a complex structure, assessing the existing factors that are part of your current situation. This includes acknowledging the logistics-only communication trap, a common pitfall for couples who prioritize efficiency over emotional engagement. Here you will gain clarity on the patterns of behavior that have led to feelings of disconnection.

By engaging with targeted exercises and prompts, you will produce your own relational metrics, enabling you to move forward with insight and hope. You will explore the emotional bandwidth of your relationship and set key connection indicators that serve as benchmarks for progress. During the DECODE Phase, you will find times and ways to connect, then scale your relationship vitality, recording this in your *Couple Connection Dashboard*. These exercises and metrics will help you systematically strengthen trust, deepen intimacy and improve communication.

ENGINEER Phase (Days 8-21)

Building on the insights gained during the DECODE Phase, in the ENGINEER Phase you will firstly set goals, then implement practical strategies to enhance your connection. Drawing on the precision and innovation side of engineering, this phase focuses on deliberate construction of new relational habits and practices. You will start using the *Couple Connection Engineering System*, a comprehensive process that empowers you to co-design your relationship to thrive.

The ENGINEER Phase centers on daily connection rituals, encouraging you to integrate these practices into your routine intentionally, just like you would with a new App or tool. By leveraging technology and structured steps, you will optimize your interactions, ensuring each moment together is richly rewarding. This is done with micro-moments, brief planned exchanges that strengthen your bond. Progressing through the ENGINEER Phase, you will track your relationship metrics using your Dashboard and scale your overall relationship vitality.

FORTIFY Phase (Days 22-28)

The culmination of your relationship renewal occurs in the FORTIFY Phase, where you secure the gains made in the preceding stages and build resilience against future challenges. Inspired by fortification and sustainability principles, this will ensure your foundations are robust enough to endure the storms of life. Here you will strategize to crisis-proof your relationship with tools that address potential stressors proactively. The

FORTIFY Phase aims for integration of your work and home roles, to support your career ambitions and relational aspirations.

Additionally, you will learn to cultivate a culture of continuous growth in your relationship, as you pursue individual and shared goals. This phase uses elements of social connection architecture, helping you to expand your support network and engage meaningfully with your community. By the end of the FORTIFY Phase, you will have increased your skills to keep your relationship thriving with strong trust, deep intimacy, and effective communication.

This three phase Couple Connection Mastery process offers a roadmap to reclaiming the loving connection that you want so much. As you engage with each phase, your relationship will grow from a state of uncertainty toward one of increasing certainty and fulfilment. This process requires commitment and intentionality, but the reward of an unbreakable bond is worth so much more than the investment you will make.

Please Note: Your 28-Day Roadmap is depicted on a Chart in Chapter Six. It has a Key for the top six metrics that you will include there, as you use it to record your progress during the 28-Days.

How to Use this Book

Throughout this action-packed workbook are practical exercises and reflection prompts I have designed to enhance your understanding and application of the principles discussed. These guide you to navigate the complexities of your relationship with confidence and clarity. I expect you to write on the charts and have added blank templates in the 'Appendices' so you can make extra copies as required. I have woven in 12 global case studies, including some cross-cultural couple stories, to portray the ways people of various nationalities are applying these skills.

As you start this rejuvenation process, remember that *Couple Connection Mastery* is not just about reaching a destination but also enjoying the growth and discovery along the way.

Closing Reflection

Sarah and Michael found it eye opening to see how their disconnection fit in the context of their family, work, and overall wellbeing. Their *Whole of System Overview* showed them how they spent their time and what led to their felt quality of life. Sarah reflected, *"This was sobering yet invaluable to see the life we have made more clearly. And to see how our mental-emotional health adds to, and results from - how well we care for our family, work and physical needs."*

Key Takeaway: Acknowledge the current state of disconnection while recognizing the potential for systematic relationship improvement.

In Chapter One, *The Partnership Drift*, we will build on this introduction with ways to recognize your connection levels and explore which love habits can make the most difference. For a printable copy of the Connection Assessment Tools in this book, see the QR Code at the end of Appendix A.

PART I

DECODE

1

THE PARTNERSHIP DRIFT

What we measure, how we measure it and how often we do this shows us what we value

— THERESE LAPPORT

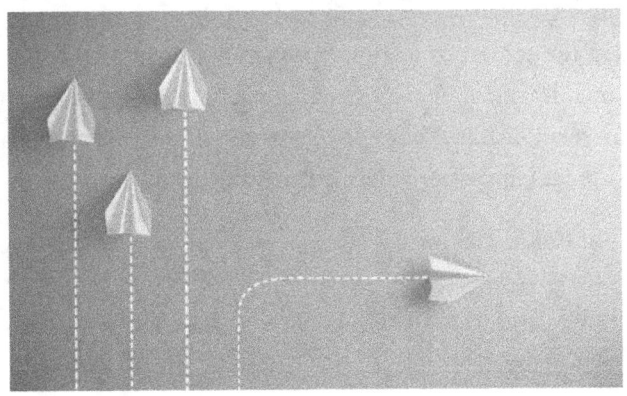

Real Life Scenario: The Morning Coffee Moment

Sarah and Michael's morning routine used to be their anchor - sharing coffee, planning their day, making small moments of connection before their work pulled them in different directions. Now, their kitchen counter resembles a command center: dueling laptops, synchronized calendars, and rapid-fire logistics about childcare and household management. Their efficiency is impressive, but something vital has slipped away in the pursuit of perfection.

"We're great business partners," Sarah confided during our first session, her voice catching slightly. *"We run this household like a well-oiled machine. But sometimes I look across the kitchen island at Michael, both of us typing away on our phones, and I wonder - when did we stop feeling really connected, heart-to-heart, and face-to-face?"*

Overview

In this chapter, you'll discover how your analytical abilities become your greatest asset in understanding relationship patterns. We address the common misconception that being analytically minded creates emotional distance - instead, we'll show how these skills provide unique advantages in relationship enhancement.

By applying the same systematic approach that drives your professional success, you'll learn to identify specific disconnection patterns that may affect your relationship. These pattern recognition skills translate vague couple challenges into clearly defined, solvable problems.

You'll try out techniques for:

- Mapping relationship dynamics with engineering precision
- Measuring current connection levels using quantifiable metrics
- Creating systematic tracking methods that fit your schedule
- Converting pattern insights into strategic action plans

This chapter is crucial to your 28-day transformation as it establishes the basis for all future improvements. Just as you wouldn't optimize a system without first understanding its current state, you'll learn to gather and analyze relationship data before implementing solutions.

By the end of this chapter, you'll have clear metrics on your current connection levels and a precise understanding of areas requiring enhancement. This data-driven foundation ensures that every future action produces measurable results, setting you up for systematic relationship improvement in the following chapters.

RECOGNIZING THE SUBTLE SIGNS OF EMOTIONAL DRIFT

Like many high-achieving couples, Sarah and Michael didn't notice their relationship shifting from intimate partnership to operational excellence.

These changes happen gradually and become evident in changes felt during daily interactions:

- That morning kiss becomes a routine peck while multi-tasking
- Date nights transform into planning sessions for home renovations
- Bedtime chats center on tomorrow's logistics rather than dreams and desires
- Physical touch becomes procedural rather than passionate
- Emotional sharing gets postponed until *"we have more time"*

With couples like this, rushing to keep up in a fast-paced industry, their days are filled with meetings and deadlines. Yet, despite winning at work, they find themselves sitting silently over dinner, conversations reduced to mere logistics about their children's schedules or the next day's to-do list. This scenario, familiar to many couples, illustrates a phenomenon known as 'partnership drift,' where the emotional connection that once thrived begins to fade into the background, overshadowed by the demands of daily life.

Recognizing the symptoms of emotional distance is crucial in addressing and reversing this drift. Often, it begins subtly with signs like those above, that can be easily overlooked. Or you find yourself withdrawing from your partner, feeling irritated by trivial things that never bothered you before, or lacking enthusiasm in conversations. These are not just fleeting moments of disconnection but can indicate an emotional gap that, if left unaddressed, may widen. Studies have shown that emotional distance can stem from high stress levels, differing emotional needs, or simply the need for more solo time, all common among high-performing individuals.

In addressing partnership drift, it is essential to pay attention to these early warning signs. A lack of affection, in words or physical touch, can be an indicator of growing distance. Similarly, disinterest in each other's daily experiences or unwillingness to work on relationship issues can further exacerbate the divide. In a healthy relationship, open communication, active listening, and mutual understanding are paramount. When these wane, the risk of emotional distance increases, leading to a fragile connection that may struggle to withstand life's pressures.

To combat these symptoms, it is vital to rebuild the attachment that initially brought you together. This involves not only improving communication but also embracing vulnerability. Sharing your feelings, fears, and aspirations with your partner can reignite the connection that may have been overshadowed by the demands of life.

UNDERSTANDING THE LOGISTICS-ONLY TRAP

In the whirlwind of daily responsibilities, it is all too easy for couples to drift into what I call the 'logistics-only trap.' This occurs when partners interact primarily through task management and coordination, focusing on schedules, errands, and endless household duties. Striving to manage these tasks well, couples may unconsciously sideline their emotional connection, reducing interactions to a series of checklists and directives. The 'logistics-only trap' can become a silent saboteur of intimacy, quietly shifting the relationship dynamic from one of close partnership to a business-like transaction, devoid of warmth and affection.

For many couples, the logistics mode becomes a default setting, driven by the necessity to organize complex lives. With children to ferry, meetings to attend, and parents to help, the focus often shifts to what must be done rather than on how partners are feeling. While efficient management is undeniably crucial, over-reliance on logistics-based conversations can erode the deeper connection that sustains relationships. This mode, left unchecked, can lead to a sense of emotional isolation, where partners feel more like co-managers than intimate allies, each performing their duties without the emotional glue that binds them together.

To illustrate, consider the typical evening of a busy couple. After a long day at work, they find themselves discussing the children's school projects, planning the week's meals, and coordinating their calendars for the next day. While this is necessary, it often leaves little room for exploring each other's emotions and needs. Over time, this can create an autopilot mode, where the relationship is maintained at a functional level but lacks the depth needed for a truly intimate partnership. In my therapy, it is common for couples caught in this trap to feel like they are unseen or unheard, with the emphasis on external tasks rather than internal experiences.

Overcoming the 'logistics-only trap' requires a conscious effort to refocus from task-oriented discussions to nurturing emotional intimacy. It involves recognizing that while logistics are a part of life, they cannot define the entirety of the relationship.

Reflection Question on Emotional Drift and the Logistics-Only Trap

Take a moment to reflect on your own relationship patterns.

When was the last time you and your partner shared a moment of genuine connection that wasn't about scheduling, planning, or problem-solving?

This is about recognition, not blame. Ironically, many couples first report *"feeling fine,"* since their partnership runs efficiently, but efficiency and intimacy are different currencies in the relationship economy. You can skilfully sync schedules while starving for emotional connection.

Exercise: The Text Connection Audit (15 minutes)

Take out your phone and review your last 20 text exchanges with your partner. Count:

- How many were purely logistical?
- How many contained emotional content?
- How many expressed appreciation or affection?
- How many were about shared dreams or future plans?

Text Topic	Contents of Our Last 20 Couple Text Messages	Stats	
Logistics	How many were purely logistical?	=	%
Emotional	How many contained emotional content?	=	%
Appreciation	How many expressed appreciation or affection?	=	%
Shared dreams	How many were about shared dreams or future plans?	=	%

This simple audit often may reveal the first concrete evidence of partnership drift.

Worked Example. Michael and Sarah – Text Connection Audit.

Text Topic	Contents of Our Last 20 Couple Text Messages	Stats
Logistics	How many were purely logistical?	14 = 70%
Emotional	How many contained emotional content?	3 = 15%
Appreciation	How many expressed appreciation or affection?	2 = 10%
Shared dreams	How many were about shared dreams or future plans?	1 = 5%

Sarah and Michael were quite shocked by their *Text Connection Audit* results, but motivated to work together to turn them around, by focusing on showing more appreciation and affection. They key was in honestly recognizing how things were first, which enabled them to assess their needs and craft micro-moments as follows below, to re-build connection.

BREAKING THE CYCLE: WITH 6-MINUTE LOVE HABITS

With Michael and Sarah, their first step of change involved tweaking their morning routine. Instead of immediately opening their laptops, they started what we call the *'6-Minute Connect.'*

The Structure of the 6-Minute Connect [Affectionately known as 6MC]

1. First 2 Minutes: Present Moment Connection
    - Make eye contact while preparing coffee
    - Share a full embrace (not a perfunctory hug)
    - Focus solely on each other - phones down
2. Middle 2 Minutes: Emotional Check-In
    - Share one hope for the day
    - Express one concern or vulnerability
    - Offer supporting acknowledgment
3. Final 2 Minutes: Appreciation and Intention
    - Express specific gratitude for something recent
    - Set one small connection intention for the day
    - End with meaningful physical contact

40 | THE PARTNERSHIP DRIFT

Remember: What we measure, how we measure it and how often - shows us what we value.

Worked Example. Michael and Sarah's 6-Minute Connect. Recorded Notes Here:

Components to Practice	Quality and Impact	Relationship Satisfaction
First 2 Minutes: Present Moment		
Make eye contact over cuppa	Ok, still waking up!	Ok
Share a full embrace	Warm and relaxing	Good
Focus together - phones away	Good to see each other	Ok / Want more
2 Minutes: Emotional Check-In		
Share one hope for the day	Ok. Hope to feel closer	Ok
Express a concern or vulnerability	Ok. Kids starting school	Ok / Anxious
Offer supporting acknowledgment	Ok. We can do this	Good
2 Minutes: Thankful & Intention		
Express gratitude for recent thing	Glad we got this book!	Good
Set connection intention for today	Lunch quick text	Hopeful
Meaningful physical contact close	Mmm - nice hug	Good
Overall – How was Your 6-Minute	**Morning Connect?** Good	**You Feel?** Bit closer

Trial Your 6-Minute Connect – And Record Your Notes Here Soon Afterward:

Components to Practice	Quality and Impact	Relationship Satisfaction
First 2 Minutes: Present Moment	*E.g Ok. Good. Helped*	*Low. Ok. Good. High. Great*
Make eye contact over cuppa		
Share a full embrace		
Focus together - phones away		
2 Minutes: Emotional Check-In		
Share one hope for the day		
Express a concern or vulnerability		
Offer supporting acknowledgment		
2 Minutes: Thankful & Intention		
Express gratitude for recent thing		
Set connection intention for today		
Meaningful physical contact		
Overall – How was Your '6-Minute	**Morning Connect?'**	**You Feel?**

THE SCIENCE BEHIND THE SHIFT

According to research, when couples engage in these structured micro-moments of connection, their physiological responses change measurably:

- Heart rates synchronize
- Stress hormones decrease
- Oxytocin levels increase
- Neural pathways associated with bonding activate

This isn't just feel-good theory - it's interpersonal neurobiological engineering for relationship success and is why '6-Minute Love Habits' work!

The 'logistics-only trap' is not an insurmountable challenge but an invitation to re-evaluate priorities and rebuild a closer partnership. By acknowledging its presence and taking deliberate steps to address it, couples can reclaim the intimacy that forms the heart of their relationship, making their connection as dynamic and fulfilling as their professional achievements.

Overcoming Common Obstacles

Some stressed disconnected couples protest, *"But we don't have 6 minutes to spare!"* And, *"Will approaches like this actually work for busy professionals like us anyway?"*

These are the most commons objection we hear. Let's address them directly.

The average person spends 5-7 minutes per hour checking their phone. We're not asking you to find more time, but to utilize your existing time better, in keeping with your couple commitment to prioritize your relationship. And yes, as you will see below, doing these exercises to assess your connection levels, then taking small, consistent actions does bring desired change.

Implementation Strategy: The 3-Day Challenge

Start small. For the next three days:

1. Set your alarm 6 minutes earlier
2. Place phones in another room during morning coffee
3. Follow the *6-Minute Connect* daily as described above
4. Document one observation about the experience each day
5. Use Chart provided or copy more from *Appendix A – Connection Assessment Tools*

Measuring Progress: Take Your Connection Baseline First

Before starting the 3-Day Challenge, establish your current baseline using these metrics:

- Number of non-logistical conversations per day
- Minutes of focused attention shared daily (no devices)
- Frequency of emotional sharing
- Instances of meaningful physical contact
- Moments of shared laughter or play

Your Couple Connection Baseline – Taken Before Your 3-Day Challenge:

Connection Method	Baseline Metrics on Top Five Couple Connection Methods	Stats
Non-logistic chats	How many of your conversations were non-logistical per day?	
Focused attention	How many minutes of focused attention (no-devices) per day?	
Emotional sharing	How often did we share emotional thoughts / feelings daily?	
Meaningful touch	How many times of affectionate physical contact per day?	
Shared playfulness	How many moments of mutual laughter or play per day?	

Worked example. Michael and Sarah - Connection Baseline.

Connection Method	Baseline Metrics on Top Five Couple Connection Methods	Stats
Non-logistic chats	How many of our conversations were non-logistical per day?	2
Focused attention	How many minutes of focused attention (no-devices) per day?	15
Emotional sharing	How often did we share emotional thoughts / feelings daily?	1
Meaningful touch	How many times of affectionate physical contact per day?	2
Shared playfulness	How many moments of mutual laughter or play per day?	1

Again, Sarah and Michael found their Connection Baseline metrics telling, but used them as a prompt for discussing how they preferred things to be. They agreed that honest assessment of how well their current system was working would help them hold onto what was ok about that, while intentionally tweaking things for gradually improving couple connection.

BREAKING THE CYCLE OF POSTPONED CONNECTION

Connecting with your partner can take a backseat in life, to the more urgent demands of work, family, and other responsibilities. The cycle of postponed connection is a subtle yet pervasive pattern where intentions to engage deeply with your partner are always deferred, awaiting *"a more convenient"* time, that rarely arrives. This cycle is not born of neglect but from the relentless tide of tasks that seem to multiply daily. For many, the belief that tomorrow, next week, or the next project will afford more time for connection is a comforting illusion, yet this mindset invariably leads to a widening emotional gulf.

Breaking this cycle requires a conscious and deliberate shift in how you perceive and prioritize your relationship. The first step is agreeing that connection cannot be relegated to the *"when there is time"* category. It must be woven into the very fabric of your daily lives. This involves integrating connection into the rhythm of your life, much like any other essential habit that sustains well-being. By treating your relationship as a dynamic entity that requires consistent attention and nurture, you can redefine what it means to be present with your partner.

Your Action Steps:

1. Complete the *Text Connection Audit* tonight
2. Share this chapter's concepts with your partner
3. Agree on a start date for the *3-Day Challenge* (to do *6MC* each morning)
4. Set up your *Connection Baseline* measurements
5. Schedule a 15-minute Weekly Check-in to discuss observations

Key Takeaway 1: Identifying relationship disconnection patterns is the first step to systematic improvement.

Understanding these patterns isn't about dwelling on problems - it's about creating a precise diagnostic in order to engineer solutions. Just as you wouldn't optimize a business without clear metrics, you can't enhance your relationship without comprehending your current patterns.

As we conclude this chapter, understand that breaking the cycle of postponed connection is an ongoing effort. It requires commitment, creativity, and willingness to prioritize your relationship amidst the myriad distractions of life. By integrating connection into the rhythms of your day, you lay the groundwork for a partnership that is not only enduring but also deeply enjoyable.

Looking Ahead: The Engineering Approach

As we progress through this program, you'll develop increasingly sophisticated connection practices. Keep in mind that everything starts with awareness and small, intentional changes.

CLOSING REFLECTION - SUCCESS STORY

Let's check on Sarah and Michael's progress. After two weeks of stops and starts trying their morning ***6-Minute Connect***, Michael reported: "We're still very efficient - we haven't lost our edge. But now there's increasing *warmth beneath the efficiency. We're feeling a bit more like connected partners again, not just co-managers."*

Success Metrics - Sarah and Michael's Updated Connection Baseline:

Connection Method	Baseline Metrics - Top Five Couple Connection Methods	Stats
Non-logistic chats	How many of our conversations were non-logistical per day?	4
Focused attention	How many minutes of focused attention (no-devices) per day?	25
Emotional sharing	How often did we share emotional thoughts/feelings daily?	2
Meaningful touch	How many times of affectionate physical contact per day?	3
Shared playfulness	How many moments of mutual laughter or play per day?	2

Michael and Sarah shared that practicing their *6-Minute Connect* each morning helped them prioritize connection at other times too, and they both felt more cared for by one another. As such, their trust, intimacy, and communication were slowly warming up.

Remember: Your journey toward unshakeable intimacy begins with this recognition phase.

In Chapter Two, *Time-Starved Love*, we'll build on this awareness to make strategic connection points throughout your day, changing time constraints from obstacles into opportunities.

2

TIME-STARVED LOVE

The most precious gift you can give your partner is time, because once spent, it can never be retrieved; invest it wisely

— UNKNOWN

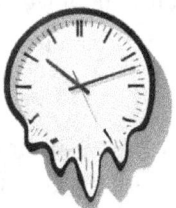

*R*eal Life Scenario: Schedule Shock in Sydney

Managing Director Alex stared at his calendar, a mosaic of stacked meetings, while his wife Jamie's surgical schedule filled their shared digital planner. *"We're both passionate about our careers,"* Alex disclosed in our coaching session, *"but last week we realized we hadn't had a decent conversation in 11 days! We'd been tracking work metrics but not relationship metrics."*

Time-Starved High-Performance Couples Like This Ask Questions Such As:

- How can we find time for connection when we're already overwhelmed?
- What's the minimum time investment needed to see tangible results?
- How do we prioritize our relationship without dropping other balls?
- Can meaningful connection really happen in just minutes per day?
- How do we make the most of the limited time we have together?

Overview

In this chapter, we'll challenge the prevailing notion that nurturing a strong relationship takes bulk leisure time – which is incompatible with a busy life. Many couples mistakenly believe that without regular, extended quality time, their connection is doomed to deteriorate. However, we'll reveal how this 'quality time myth' can hinder rather than help your relationship.

Instead, you'll discover the relational power of *'engineered micro-moments'* - brief, intentional experiences that foster intimacy and understanding. We'll explore how to strategically design these moments to fit smoothly into your day, so your bond becomes vibrant and strong. This is what we call *'relating smarter, not harder.'*

Using practical examples and actionable strategies, we will equip you to start renewing your connection without overhauling your entire schedule. You'll learn how to optimize small pockets of time, infuse interactions with meaning, and create rituals that keep you emotionally attuned.

By the end of this chapter, you will have mapped your connection points and tried out proven techniques to cultivate closeness, no matter how hectic life is. Get ready to revolutionize the way you think about quality time and unlock the power of strategic micro-connections. Your strongest, most fulfilling partnership awaits.

DEBUNKING THE QUALITY TIME MYTH

Let's address the elephant in the room - the well-meaning but misguided application of *"just making more quality time."* The original idea is adapted from Dr Gary Chapman's brilliant insights on the Five Love Languages, how we learn to feel loved by receiving acts of service, affirming words, affectionate touch, gifts, or quality time with caregivers. Those with quality time as their primary love language will feel more loved when they have longer time with close others.

However, this is likely true for only one in five people, as the other 80% will have gifts, touch, words, or kind actions as their primary love language. Dr Chapman *never asserted that everyone would feel loved by the length of quality time they spend with their closest people*, but instead - by receiving love that is intentionally communicated on their love language frequency.

However, much traditional relationship guidance still assumes the following will be possible:

- Weekly date nights
- Weekend getaways
- Long intimate conversations

For high-performing couples, these may create more stress than solutions. Here's why.

The Reality of Modern Partnership

Looking back at our *'Whole of System Assessment'* in the introductory chapter, review your:

- Hours spent at work and commuting
- Family obligations
- Essential self-care
- Sleep requirements

In that exercise, you assessed your time use and quality of life. The math is clear - with tight timeframes, there isn't a hidden reservoir of 'quality time' waiting to be discovered. We need a smarter approach that leverages our time better. In the lives of high-achieving couples, the notion of 'quality time' may be presented as a panacea for relationship woes. The belief that big chunks of planned time together compensate for the lack of small everyday interactions.

Yet, this concept, while comforting, does not address how real couples meet their genuine need for connection and intimacy. With schedules packed to the brim, they may cling to the hope that a monthly date night, meticulously orchestrated, will bridge the growing emotional gap. However, when the evening arrives, the weight of unspoken frustrations and accumulated exhaustion can overshadow their intentions, leaving them unfulfilled and disconnected.

The reality for many high-performing couples is that their lives are dictated by ticking clocks and tight deadlines, leaving little room for long leisurely hours to foster meaningful connection. In such scenarios, the pressure to make every moment count can back fire, turning a simple activity into a performance where the focus shifts from enjoying each other's company to fulfilling an expectation of what 'quality time' should entail. This manufactured pressure can create a cycle of disappointment, where attempts to connect feel inadequate, further alienating partners who are already strained by their myriad responsibilities.

To debunk the quality time myth, it is imperative to recognize that meaningful connection is not confined to grand gestures or meticulously planned outings. Instead, it is woven, 'little and often,' into the mundane fabric of daily life, in quiet moments over morning coffee or the shared laughter during a quick lunch break. These seemingly insignificant interactions can hold the greatest potential for closeness, as they occur naturally and without the burden of expectation.

By shifting the focus from quantity to quality in its truest sense, couples can find fulfilment in the everyday exchanges that sustain their relationships.

This perspective invites a re-evaluation of how time is utilized, encouraging couples to prioritize presence over perfection. It means accepting that connection is a continuous process, not a destination to be reached through rare instances of togetherness. Integrating connection into your routine by acts as simple as a heartfelt text or shared moments of reflection before sleep, helps couples like you to nurture a bond that withstands the pressures of life.

This approach transforms the narrative from one of scarcity - where time is a limited resource to be hoarded - into one of abundance, where each moment holds the potential for connection.

Note: For those who enjoy quality time as their primary love language, the above does not negate this. It clarifies the need *to plan how to express love languages effectively within time limits.* Couple connection can of course be boosted through date nights, couple therapy and getaways - if suited to your lifestyle. Like most wisdom, it's not 'either-or,' but 'both-and,' based on the quality and quantity of time you need together. Hence, we focus here on how to prioritize your relationship by systematically engineering connection within your schedules.

THE POWER OF MICRO-MOMENTS FOR ENGINEERING CONNECTION

In the demanding workaday world, where every minute seems accounted for, micro-moments offer a refreshing perspective on how connections can be nurtured without the luxury of expansive time. These micro-moments are brief yet meaningful interactions that happen intentionally, offering profound opportunities for connection amid hectic schedules.

Take the example of our couple - Alex the MD and Jamie the surgeon - both working in high-stakes environments. Despite their demanding careers, they found ways to interject micro-moments of connection throughout their day. A quick but sincere voice message, or a moment of laughter invoked by a text during a morning routine - such small gestures are deceptively powerful. They serve as anchors that keep you connected, even when time is tight.

Micro-moments thrive on the principle of presence. They require you to be fully engaged, even if just for a few seconds, acknowledging the importance of your partner. This approach challenges the notion that meaningful interactions require large blocks of dedicated time. Instead, it highlights the significance of quality small exchanges. The beauty of micro-moments lies in their accessibility; they can happen anytime, anywhere. Whether it's a reassuring touch on the arm while passing each other in the hallway or a shared smile over a mundane task, these moments accumulate, thickening connection that enriches your relationship.

The effectiveness of micro-moments is rooted in their ability to foster positivity resonance, a term coined by psychologist Barbara Fredrickson. This concept depicts the synchronization of positive emotions between individuals, leading to a shared sense of connection and upliftment.

In relationships, micro-moments are building blocks of positivity resonance. They create an emotional feedback loop, reinforcing the bond between partners through shared joy, empathy, and understanding. By consciously engineering these moments, you can make an environment where positive emotions flourish, incrementally strengthening your relationship.

For high-achieving couples, their challenge often lies in recognizing and seizing these micro-moments amidst daily responsibilities. *It requires a shift in mindset, where you see interactions not as interruptions but as opportunities to connect.*

This view urges you to remain attentive and responsive to your partner's bids for connection, acknowledging their presence and importance in your life. These moments are not big or flashy but subtle, often unspoken expressions of love and commitment. By valuing these interactions, you prioritize your relationship in a way that transcends time constraints.

THE SCIENCE OF MICRO-CONNECTION

Research shows that multiple brief, intentional connections throughout the day can be more powerful than occasional longer periods of time together. This is because they:

- Maintain emotional attunement
- Reduce stress accumulation
- Create ongoing safety signals
- Build relationship resilience

The global validity of intentional brief, regular habits is well established and applied in various dimensions of wellbeing. These range from physical acts like hydration and postural micro-pauses for muscle relaxation, to self-calming like Mindfulness Based Stress Reduction (MBSR), or spiritual practices of contemplative centring prayer like The Daily Office.

Physical workout options like High Intensity Interval training (HIIT) or muscular exercise principles like TUT – Time Under Tension are well known examples. As recent studies have shown, the same timeless principle applies in all facets of wellbeing including relational, parental, work and financial. The best fruit or 'return on investment' comes from micro-habits practiced 'little and often.' Consistency is the key, hence our systematic focus.

Exercise: Best Connection Point Mapping - Discovering Your BCPs (10 minutes)

1. List your daily transition points
2. Identify existing touch points
3. Note current missed opportunities
4. Mark potential new connection moments

With Jamie and Alex, this Connection Point Mapping exercise helped them find opportunities and set about creatively utilizing those moments. By Mapping, they discovered what we call *'Best Connection Points'* (BCPs) within their daily timetables.

1. Transition Moments (30 seconds)
    - Arriving home greetings
    - Leaving for work rituals
    - Shift changes in parenting duties
2. Digital Touch Points (1 minute)
    - Strategic message timing
    - Emotional shorthand use
    - Priority flagging system
3. Parallel Activity Connection (ongoing)
    - Working side by side with periodic check-ins
    - Physically exercising together
    - Sharing morning routines

Implementation Strategy: Using Daily 'BCPs' to Do More 6 Minute Connects

After a week's satisfactory results trying connection methods at their mapped daily points, Alex and Jamie felt encouraged, so they specifically adapted their *6MC* use into this plan:

Morning Launch Sequence (3 minutes)

- 60-second physical connection
- 60-second emotional check-in
- 60-second intention setting

Daytime Digital Bridge (30 seconds each)

- Three pre-scheduled message times
- Specific emotional content focus
- No logistics allowed

Evening Reconnection Ritual (3 minutes)

- 60-second full attention greeting
- 60-second stress release support
- 60-second gratitude exchange

See their results Charted below.

STRATEGIC CONNECTION IN A BUSY WORLD

Finding meaningful connection with your partner can feel like a daunting task. High-performing people find their days filled with work and constantly humming digital notifications. *This is why your analytical abilities must be used to build connection intentionally and strategically.* The key lies in integrating connection into the fabric of your daily routine, ensuring it becomes a natural and indispensable part of your life.

Consider the concept of strategic connection as akin to a well-executed business plan. Just as you prioritize tasks that align with your professional goals, you must also prioritize interactions that enhance your relationship. This involves a deliberate commitment to carve out time, even in the busiest schedules, for interactions that foster understanding and emotional closeness. By treating these moments as non-negotiable appointments, you reinforce the importance of your relationship, ensuring it receives the attention it deserves.

Your Implementation Plan: Map and Utilize BCPs for Connection and Learning

1. Today
    - Complete *Connection Point Mapping*
    - Identify three potential BCPs
    - Plan to discuss action steps
2. This Week
    - Choose one BCP to implement
    - Design specific protocol
    - Use the recording Chart
3. This Fortnight
    - Add two more BCPs
    - Refine timing and approach
    - Document impact and adjustment

Measuring Success: Key Metrics

Once you've Mapped them, try out tracking your *BCP* metrics daily (Jamie & Alex used Phone Notes – but you can write below in the Chart provided):

- Number of successful BCPs
- Quality of each connection
- Impact on emotional state
- Effect on relationship satisfaction

Recording a Trial Week of Utilizing BCPs for Connection and Learning:

Daily Number of Successful BCPs	Average Quality of Each BCP Connection	Impact on Emotional State of Both Partners	Effect on Relationship Satisfaction Reported
Monday =			
Tuesday =			
Wednesday =			
Thursday =			
Friday =			
Saturday =			
Sunday =			
Average = /Day	Quality =		

Real-World Application: Success Story

After Jamie and Alex's first seven days of practicing these strategies, they achieved:

- Morning connection protocol: 3 minutes on average per day
- Daytime digital check-ins: 2 x 30 seconds average daily
- Evening reconnection: 3 minutes on average.
- Total daily investment = 7 minutes.

Success Metrics - Jamie and Alex's First 7 Days using BCPs for Connection and Learning:

Number of Daily Successful BCPs	Average Quality of Each BCP Connection	Impact on Emotional State of Both Partners	Effect on Relationship Satisfaction Reported
Monday = 3	Ok - Good	Felt warmer	Up a little
Tuesday = 4	Good	Closer	Improved
Wednesday = 4	Ok - Good	Glad doing this	Good & thankful
Thursday = 4	Good	Warmer	Stronger
Friday = 4	Better	Closer	Higher
Saturday = 4	Good - moderate	Relaxed & happier	Positive
Sunday = 5 T = 28	Moderate - high	Grateful to be closer	Boosted
Average = 4/Day	Quality = Good+	Warmer & Closer	**Raised Satisfaction**

Reported relationship satisfaction increase compared with a week earlier: 16%

Key Takeaway 2: Meaningful connection can be achieved through strategically designed brief interactions.

Success isn't about finding more time - but engineering your time for the best benefits. We all get 86,400 seconds per day. Each moment contains the potential for deepening your connection.

CLOSING REFLECTION

Alex and Jamie's story continues: "We stopped waiting for the perfect moment and started creating perfect moments within our everyday reality. Our connection feels a bit closer and more consistent now, even though we're just as busy. It's about intention, not duration."

Remember: You don't need to overhaul your schedule to renew your relationship. You just need to engineer the moments you already have. If your top two love languages include quality time, it will be even more important to optimize the quality of the time you share.

In Chapter 3, *The Science of Connection*, we'll explore how to measure and track these connection points, creating a data-driven approach to relationship improvement. You'll learn to use metrics not just for your career, but for your most important partnership.

3

THE SCIENCE OF CONNECTION

Neurons that fire together, wire together

— DONALD HEBB

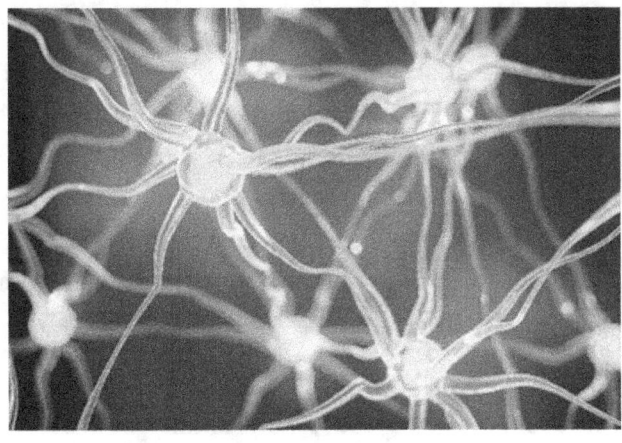

Real Life Scenario: Bedtime Breaking Point in Britain

"I used to love our bedtime routine," Lisa confided, glancing at her partner Richard, who nodded in agreement. "Now it's just tactical warfare - getting three kids bathed, storied, and settled while answering work emails and trying not to snap at each other. By the time we crawl into bed, we're too exhausted to even hold hands, let alone be intimate."

This London based couple in their thirties, were tired out. By day Lisa project managed teams of electrical engineers, while Richard was a senior legal partner in a conveyancing firm. Richard added softly, *"The other night, one of our 5-year-old twins asked why we don't kiss like we used to. That hit hard. We're teaching them about relationships by default, aren't we?"*

Disconnected High-Performance Couples Often Ask Questions Like These:

- How do we measure our current connection level?
- What specific behaviors are damaging our bond?
- Which areas of our relationship need the most attention?

Overview

Under every strong relationship lies a foundation of measurable patterns and trackable growth points. For high-achieving professionals who thrive on data-driven decisions, understanding these patterns decodes relationship building from a mysterious art into a precise science. This chapter bridges the gap between emotional intelligence and quantifiable metrics, showing you how to apply your analytical strengths to relationship development.

The science of connection isn't about reducing your relationship to cold numbers - it's about leveraging your natural affinity for measurement and analysis to strengthen your emotional bonds. Just as you track KPIs in your professional work, you'll learn to identify and monitor the key indicators of your relationship health, transforming abstract concepts like 'feeling connected' into concrete, measurable scores called *Key Connection Indicators* or *'KCIs.'*

By applying the same analytical rigor to your relationship as you use in your work roles, you will:

- Translate subjective feelings into measurable data points
- Create systematic approaches to tracking relationship vitality
- Develop clear metrics for measuring progress

This chapter provides the scientific metrics required for your future relationship engineering work, guiding your path to deeper connection with clear information, rather than guesswork.

UNDERSTANDING EMOTIONAL BANDWIDTH

The science of connection isn't just about time management, but also energy allocation. When your toddler's having their third tantrum today, your teenager's stressed with school drama, and you've both got critical work deadlines - emotional and physical intimacy can feel too hard. But the truth is - meaningful connection isn't 'just another task on the list,' - it's the fuel making everything else possible. Couple connection must be top priority to thrive under pressure.

In the fast-paced and demanding world of high-achievers, understanding the intricacies of emotional bandwidth is necessary for fostering a deeply connected relationship. Picture a couple, thriving in their careers, yet finding themselves emotionally drained at the end of the day, unable to truly engage with one another. This scenario is common, as the stresses of life often stretch our emotional capacities to their limits, leaving little room for connection.

Your emotional bandwidth means your ability to manage and respond to emotional stimuli, and is a key factor in the quality of your interactions with loved ones. It encompasses emotional resilience and intelligence, plus the capacity to navigate emotionally challenging situations with grace and empathy. High emotional bandwidth enables individuals to connect deeply with their partners, effectively resolve conflicts, and maintain psychological resilience amidst stress.

Understanding emotional bandwidth starts with realizing its dynamic nature. It fluctuates based on factors like stress and energy levels, and mental wellness. When emotional bandwidth is high, individuals can manage relationship complexities with ease, deepening connections and communicating effectively. However, when it is low, feelings of emotional depletion, overwhelm and fatigue can arise, impacting all dimensions of wellbeing. Recognizing the signs of stretched emotional bandwidth is essential for maintaining emotional health and ensuring the vitality of your relationship. Symptoms like irritability, emotional exhaustion, and difficulty concentrating can serve as indicators that your emotional capacity is nearing its limits.

To enhance emotional bandwidth, do simple acts of self-care and engage in practices that promote emotional intelligence and being present. These can replenish emotional reserves, enabling you to engage more fully with your partner. Mindfulness, in particular, offers a powerful way to expand emotional bandwidth by cultivating present-moment awareness and reducing stress. It involves paying attention to thoughts and emotions without judgment, allowing for a greater understanding of one's emotional landscape. By incorporating brief mindful practices into your daily routine, you can increase emotional resilience and enhance your capacity to connect with your partner. These practices can be a part of your *6MC* love habits.

MEASURING RELATIONSHIP VITALITY

In the rugged terrain of today's relationships, checking the vitality of your partnership is crucial. Measuring relationship vitality goes beyond the superficial markers of success, delving into the subtler aspects of your connection. Imagine your relationship as a living organism requiring regular checkups to ensure its health and longevity. Just as you monitor your physical health through regular exams, or your car via regular safety checks, your relationship vitality must be evaluated to show its strengths and needs. This involves qualitative and quantitative measures, allowing you to capture a comprehensive picture of your partnership's resilience and vibrancy.

Creating Your Key Connection Indicators = KCIs

Key Connection Indicators or *KCIs*, help you understand and enhance your relationship, like a snapshot of your current relational state, offering insight into your emotional, psychological, and behavioral patterns. These KCIs give you a reference point from which growth and change can be measured. Like a business relies on metrics to gauge success and identify areas for improvement, your relationship benefits from a similar approach. Identifying where you stand, gives you clarity on the strengths to nurture and the issues to address.

Creating *Key Connection Indicators* is not a 'once-and-done,' but an ongoing process. As your relationship evolves, your KCIs will too, adapting to new experiences, trials and aspirations. We will regularly revisit your KCIs, updating them to reflect current realities and future hopes. This practice reinforces the notion that relationships are dynamic, requiring continuous attention and adaptation. By embracing this iterative process, you can cultivate your relationship to stay responsive to change, robust in the face of adversity, and enriched by shared growth.

As you establish your KCIs, consider the wider context of your individual and collective goals, as we did in the *Whole of System Overview* earlier. *How do your personal ambitions align with your relationship trajectory? In what areas can you support each other's growth while maintaining a strong partnership?* These questions invite deeper exploration, encouraging a holistic view of your relationship's role in your life. By integrating your *Key Connection Indicators* with your life objectives, you create a cohesive narrative that honors both individual and collective goals.

The question Lisa and Richard raised, *"What does healthy connection look like for busy couples with young children?"* requires specific action suited to your context. Healthy connection must incorporate the daily physical, emotional and mental ways you engage with each other and your children if you have them - or with other generations of family members and relatives.

Like monitoring your children's growth charts or your quarterly business metrics, we'll track key indicators of your couple connection below. These are the *Key Connection Indicators* of your *Relationship Vitality*. A *KCIs Metrics* chart is provided below for you to use.

1. **Physical Connection Metrics**
   - Daily affectionate touches
   - Non-sexual physical affection
   - Sleep proximity patterns
   - Sexually intimate moments
2. **Emotional Connection Metrics**
   - Deep conversations initiated
   - Vulnerable shares exchanged
   - Supportive moments offered
   - Joint parenting wins celebrated
3. **Mental Connection Metrics**
   - Shared decisions made
   - Problems solved together
   - Future plans discussed
   - Parenting strategies aligned

Your Connection KCIs – Record Your Metrics & Experiences Here:

THREE TYPES OF CONNECTION	Quantity and Quality	Relationship Satisfaction
Physical Connection Metrics	*E.g 1-2. Ok. Good. Helped*	*Low. Good. High. Great*
Daily affectionate touches		
Non-sexual physical affection		
Sleep proximity patterns		
Sexually intimate moments		
Emotional Connection Metrics		
Deep conversations initiated		
Vulnerable shares exchanged		
Supportive moments offered		
Joint parenting wins		
Mental Connection Metrics		
Shared decisions made		
Problems solved together		
Future plans discussed		
Parenting strategies aligned		
Overall: How is Your Three-Fold	Connection?	You Feel?

Couple Case Study Example: The Reconnection Journey

With Lisa and Richard, parents of three under eight:

- Initial state: *"Ships passing in the night"*
- Key challenge: Constant childcare demands
- Hidden issue: Growing resentment over division of labor
- Core need: Rebuilding physical and emotional intimacy

66 | THE SCIENCE OF CONNECTION

Worked Example - Lisa and Richard's Connection KCIs and Notes

THREE TYPES OF CONNECTION	Quantity and Quality	Relationship Satisfaction
Physical Connection Metrics		
Daily affectionate touches	2. Ok	Low
Non-sexual physical embraces	1. Good	Ok
Sleep proximity patterns	6 Hours. Same bed. Ok	Ok
Sexually intimate moments	Once this week. Ok	Good
Emotional Connection Metrics		
Deep conversations initiated	1. Ok	Low
Vulnerable shares exchanged	No - too tired	Ok
Supportive moments offered	1 or 2	Good
Joint parenting wins	1	Ok. Need more
Mental Connection Metrics		
Shared decisions made	Lots about kids	Ok
Problems solved together	2. About kids and bills	Ok
Future plans discussed	1. Short term e.g weekend	Low
Parenting strategies aligned	Helping each other more	Ok
Overall: How is Your Three-Fold	**Connection?** Bit warmer	**You Feel?** Tired. Hopeful

After a week of paying attention to their connection metrics like this, Lisa and Richard crafted the following tailored approach. They called it: The *'Partners First, Parents Always'* Protocol

Morning Connection (Pre-Kids Wake-Up)

- 5:30-45 AM: Sacred coffee time
- Physical affection priority
- No phones, no planning
- Just being present together

Day-Time Bridging

- Friendly text window (10-10:30 AM)
- Lunch break check-in
- Parenting win celebrations
- *"I see you"* moments

Evening Recovery

- Kids' bedtime teamwork
- 10-minute reconnection ritual
- Intimate space creation
- Permission to be imperfect

For Lisa and Richard, intentionally prioritizing their couple connection did not create new time each day, but it helped them pull together deliberately as a team. See their progress further down, after recording your final metrics and constructing your *Relationship Dashboard*.

Scaling Trust, Intimacy and Communication in Light of Your Metrics Above

Review your recorded Metrics above, then with your partner, rate the resulting quality of these three core connection ingredients on our **Trust, Intimacy and Communication Scale (TICS)**

Trust Scale: 0 _____ 10 (10 = Best)

Intimacy Scale: 0 _____ 10

Communication Scale: 0 _____ 10

Now Combine your Metrics, Connection KCIs and TIC Scale to Rate Your Resulting:

RELATIONSHIP VITALITY SCALE: 0 _____ 10 (10 = Best)

How does the rating you gave here seem to you, taking all your metrics into account? Now does it make sense that we have used quantifiable metrics to measure the quality of your connection?

RELATIONSHIP VITALITY DASHBOARD FOR COUPLE CONNECTION MASTERY

Having assessed your relationship vitality, let's bring your top seven metrics together in one place where you can see them in a one-stop-shop

Relationship Dashboard. This Dashboard helps you view the key parts of your connection, to appreciate, assess and improve them.

1. **The Text Connection Audit** (15 minutes)

Text Topic	Contents of Our Last 20 Couple Text Messages	Stats	
Logistics	How many were purely logistical?	=	%
Emotional	How many contained emotional content?	=	%
Appreciation	How many expressed appreciation or affection?	=	%
Shared dreams	How many were about shared dreams or future plans?	=	%

2. **Your 6-Minute Connect Trial - Record Your Notes Here:**

Components to Practice	Quality and Impact	Relationship Satisfaction
First 2 Minutes: Present Moment	E.g Ok. Good. Helped	Low. Ok. Good. High. Great
Make eye contact over cuppa		
Share a full embrace		
Focus together - phones away		
2 Minutes: Emotional Check-In		
Share one hope for the day		
Express a concern or vulnerability		
Offer supporting acknowledgment		
2 Minutes: Thankful & Intention		
Express gratitude for recent thing		
Set connection intention for today		
Meaningful physical contact		
Overall – How was Your '6-Minute	Morning Connect?'	You Feel?

3. **Connection Baseline – Taken Before Your 3-Day Challenge:**

Connection Method	Baseline Metrics on Top Five Couple Connection Methods	Stats
Non-logistic chats	How many of your conversations were non-logistical per day?	
Focused attention	How many minutes of focused attention (no-devices) per day?	
Emotional sharing	How often did we share emotional thoughts / feelings daily?	
Meaningful touch	How many times of affectionate physical contact per day?	
Shared playfulness	How many moments of mutual laughter or play per day?	

4. Utilizing BCPs - Record of Trial Week for Connection and Learning:

Daily Number of Successful BCPs	Average Quality of Each BCP Connection	Impact on Emotional State of Both Partners	Effect on Relationship Satisfaction Reported
Monday =			
Tuesday =			
Wednesday =			
Thursday =			
Friday =			
Saturday =			
Sunday =			
Average = /Day	Quality =		

5. Connection KCIs – Record Your Metrics & Experiences Here:

THREE TYPES OF CONNECTION	Quantity and Quality	Relationship Satisfaction
Physical Connection Metrics	*E.g 1-2. Ok. Good. Helped*	*Low. Good. High. Great*
Daily affectionate touches		
Non-sexual physical affection		
Sleep proximity patterns		
Sexually intimate moments		
Emotional Connection Metrics		
Deep conversations initiated		
Vulnerable shares exchanged		
Supportive moments offered		
Joint parenting wins		
Mental Connection Metrics		
Shared decisions made		
Problems solved together		
Future plans discussed		
Parenting strategies aligned		
Overall: How is Your Three-Fold	Connection?	You Feel?

6. Scaling Trust, Intimacy and Communication in Light of Your Metrics Above

Review your recorded Metrics above, then Rate with your partner the resulting quality of these three connection ingredients on our: **Trust, Intimacy and Communication Scale (TICS).** Note: it is normal for partners to give different ratings on these connection vital signs - for discussion.

Trust Scale: 0 _____ 10 (10 = Best)

Intimacy Scale: 0 _____ 10

Communication Scale: 0 _____ 10

7. Combine your Metrics, Connection KCIs and TIC Scale to Rate Your Resulting

RELATIONSHIP VITALITY SCALE: 0 _____ **10** (10 = Best)

The Science Behind 'Partner-Parent Balance'

Research shows that couples with strong intimate connections:

- Manage parenting stress better
- Present more unified fronts
- Raise more secure children
- Maintain relationship satisfaction

Success Story: Lisa and Richard's Transformation

Three weeks into implementing their connection metrics, measuring and tracking them:

- Morning intimacy increased 15%
- Parenting conflicts decreased 27%
- Physical affection doubled
- Children noticed and commented positively

Richard affirmed that their key insight was: *"When we prioritize our connec-*

tion first, we're warmer, closer and naturally better parents. The kids sense it, and everyone benefits."

Your Action Steps

1. Today
    - Complete *TIC Scale*
    - Scale *Relationship Vitality*
    - Schedule implementation discussion
2. This Week
    - Start tracking on this *Relationship Dashboard*
    - Create measurement routine
    - Continue data collection
3. This Month
    - Review and adjust metrics
    - Celebrate improvements
    - Refine approach based on data

Key Takeaway 3: Quantifiable metrics enable systematic relationship improvement. Under-standing your connection patterns with this data helps transform abstract goals into achievable actions, even amid the beautiful chaos of family life.

CLOSING REFLECTION

"Last night," Lisa shared in our follow-up session, "*we had to pause three times during our physical intimacy for various kids' needs. Instead of getting frustrated though, we laughed. We've learned to surf the interruptions instead of fighting them. Our connection is stronger because it's real - dealing with kids' toilet and sleep issues, Lego landmines, and all.*"

Remember: Perfect conditions never come. Grow connection in your beautiful, messy reality.

In Chapter Four, *Engineering Love*, we'll explain the Couple Connection Engineering System, centered around the Relationship BUILD Framework and incorporating the metrics we already have. This 28-Day Roadmap will help you plan realistic connection goals, implement action steps, record progress, regularly review and optimize your system for sustainability.

4

ENGINEERING LOVE

At its heart, engineering is using science to find creative practical solutions. It is a noble profession

— QUEEN ELIZABETH

Real Life Scenario: The Minivan Moment in Massachusetts

Boston-based Maya, a senior Information Systems Analyst, and her husband Marcus - a Chief Technology Officer, described the discrepancies between their professional skills and the state of their marriage and family, highlighting a recent situation that brought things to a head.

"It hit me in the minivan," Marcus laughed, explaining during our session. "Maya and I were tag teaming - she's passing snacks to the girls, I'm mediating a Minecraft dispute with our 8-year-old, both our phones are dinging with work messages, and suddenly I realized - we've got engineering degrees from MIT, we design systems for a living but have never applied that mindset to our relationship!?"

Maya nodded, bouncing their youngest on her lap. "We were optimizing everything except us. Our kids had detailed schedules, our work had clear KPIs, but our intimacy? Complete chaos."

High-Performance Couples with Chaotic Parenting and Work Lives Often Ask:

- What does healthy connection look like for busy couples who are parents?
- How do we know if we're making progress in our relationship?

Overview

Generic relationship advice must be adapted for analytical high-achievers, or it can miss their natural inclination toward systematic improvement and measurable progress.

This chapter introduces the Couple Connection Engineering System, central to which is the Relationship BUILD Framework - *specifically designed for professionals who excel at optimizing complex systems but struggle with applying those skills to emotional connection.*

The Relationship BUILD Framework isn't just another theory - *it's a precision-engineered* methodology *that aligns with how high-performance couples naturally think and operate.* By treating relationship enhancement as a system optimization challenge, you'll discover how to apply your professional strengths to personal connection. *This renewal happens, not by making big changes, but through strategically designed micro-improvements that compound over time.*

Your professional success comes from your ability to break down complex challenges into manageable bite-sized chunks. Now you'll learn to:

- Apply systems thinking to relationship development
- Transform abstract emotional goals into concrete action steps
- Create measurable checkpoints for relationship progress
- Design efficient processes for emotional connection

This chapter establishes the plan for your 28-day transformation journey, providing the blueprint for engineering unshakeable love through precise, measurable steps that respect your time constraints and leverage your analytical strengths.

INTRODUCING THE COUPLE CONNECTION ENGINEERING SYSTEM

Marcus and Maya were peaking in their bustling careers in IT, where innovation and efficiency reigned, but not at applying strategic planning to their relationship and parenting.

For many high-performing couples, the notion of engineering love might seem unconventional, yet it offers a pragmatic approach to nurturing a thriving partnership. This chapter presents the *Couple Connection Engineering System*, a process designed to infuse your relationship with the same intentionality and foresight that drives your professional success.

At the heart of this system lies the belief that relationships, like any successful enterprise, are built on solid understanding, trust, and shared vision. By linking concepts from the strategic processes in the tech industry and the dynamics of a relationship, I created a comprehensive blueprint for love that is innovative and enduring. *The Couple Connection Engineering System* leverages engineering principles, emotional intelligence, and practical strategies to guide couples in constructing a relationship that is durable and deeply fulfilling.

The Relationship BUILD Framework

This provides a strategic pathway for couples to enhance their connection. It offers a roadmap that aligns with the realities of life and the demands placed on high-achievers, by providing practical steps to prioritize and nurture their partnership. By following this framework, couples can create a resilient, loving relationship that mirrors their success in other areas of life.

In technology and engineering, frameworks act as scaffolding upon which complex systems are built - giving structure, clarity, and direction. *The Relationship BUILD Framework* provides a structured way to strengthen your connection. The process of relationship enhancement is chunked into five key phases: Base; Understand; Implement; Leverage; and Deepen. Together, these form a step-by-step guide that helps couples to align their relationship and work success.

The first phase is BASE. Just as skyscrapers require deep underpinning to support their towering height, a relationship needs a well-defined base. This phase involves establishing metrics for the connection levels in your relationship. Then, by aligning your goals, you create a sense of unity and direction as you strengthen your bond.

The **UNDERSTAND phase** prompts you to find the best connection points in your daily schedules. It's about understanding patterns and opportunities for connection, and what helps achieve that. It also looks at what triggers you or your partner, and how this damages your connection, then what helps you to recover from that. When partners take time to truly connect and comprehend each other, their bond feels both profoundly safe and enduringly strong.

In the IMPLEMENT phase, you enact the insights from prior stages to *practice morning rituals* that build your connection. You will use the love habits introduced earlier, implementing those with *6MCs* at connection points mapped when you did your *BCPs*. You then add *Midday Check-ins* to your morning connections. The key is consistency and employing these love habits will ensure your relationship stays top priority in your daily responsibilities.

After this, **the LEVERAGE phase** prompts you to capitalize on the strengths of your relationship. Here you salute and celebrate your successes, big and small, using them as a springboard for further growth, including *evening connection habits*. Leveraging involves pattern refinement and strategy scaling as you utilize your skills to benefit your partnership. By maximizing these strengths, you will create a dynamic that is greater than the sum of its parts.

Finally, **the DEEPEN phase** helps you integrate your love habits into strong routines so that your relationship flourishes long-term. You will cultivate a deeper emotional connection with practice and maintenance of your connection routines. This phase reinforces the idea that a relationship is not static but is an evolving entity that blossoms with time and effort.

YOUR 28-DAY TRANSFORMATION ROADMAP TO BETTER CONNECTION:

As you stand ready to embark on your relationship renewal, *envision the 28-day transformation roadmap as a meticulously crafted itinerary. Over these coming four weeks, each day serves as a stepping stone to a more connected and harmonious partnership.* This roadmap is your guide through the process, offering a structured approach to practices that support lasting change. It is designed to be adapted to the intricacies of your lives, so each day contributes meaningfully to your relationship's growth, without overwhelming your schedule. Record your metrics from here on in your 28-Day Roadmap Progress Chart, provided to be written on, in Chapter Six.

WEEK ONE focuses on evaluation and understanding. You will do activities to assess the current state of your relationship, identifying strengths and areas needing attention. This week is about clarity that sets the stage for the work to come. You will dialogue with your partner about your shared goals and *practice morning connection*. This foundational work is crucial to aligning your intentions and ensuring both partners are committed to the process. By the end of week one, you will have a clear understanding of where you are and where you plan to go.

In the WEEK TWO, you will implement new love habits. Inspired by the insights gained in week one, you will *introduce midday habits* to your routine. These will build connection and intimacy. This week will involve time for checking what habits bring you closer. The emphasis is on consistency and intentionality, ensuring these practices become integral to your relationship. By mid-week, you should start to notice a shift in your dynamics, with increased communication and understanding forming the bedrock of your partnership.

During WEEK THREE, you will start optimization and refinement. Building on the habits you established earlier, you will fine-tune your approach, so your changes are sustainable and effective. In this week you will *adopt evening connection habits* and check how these affect your family system. Strategic practice, whilst staying adaptable and open, will make your growth a continuous process. By the end of week three, you should find that your relationship feels more cohesive and aligned, with a renewed sense of purpose guiding your interactions.

WEEK FOUR of the roadmap is dedicated to consolidation and celebration of the progress you have made, acknowledging the growth and changes that have occurred over the past month. You are encouraged to honor your achievements, individually and as a couple, recognizing the effort and commitment that has brought you to this point. This week also invites you to craft the next steps in your relationship's development, setting intentions for the future and identifying areas for further growth. The aim is that the advancements you have made are not only sustained, but continue to flourish in the months and years to come.

As this chapter ends, you can now see how we will use this sequential roadmap to guide the renewal of your relationship. This 28-day process will provide the structure and support to make your partnership as successful and fulfilling as your careers are. The principles and practices you apply will enable your relationship to thrive amidst the complexities and demands of life.

Like Marcus and Maya, many high-achieving parents excel at systems thinking everywhere except their relationship. They chose to change that by going through the prior exercises to find their *Best Connection Points (BCPs)* then doing **6-Minute Connect** in their mornings.

CLOSING REFLECTION - SUCCESS STORY

As Maya and Marcus shared, *"We used to collapse into weekend survival mode. Now we have our 'Connection Command Center'- our Relationship Vitality Dashboard - where we track our Key Connection Indicators, plus our Trust, Intimacy and Communication metrics, in one place. Now we have a better grasp of our relationship system, we can think when it might work best to try and make kid-free moments that work with our daily energy patterns."*

The Science of System Success

Research shows engineered approaches succeed because:

- Clear metrics drive behavior
- Systems beat willpower
- Protocols reduce decision fatigue
- Measurement enables improvement

Key Takeaway 4: A systematic approach transforms relationship improvement from over-whelming to achievable.

Real Results: Marcus and Maya's Update

Three weeks later: *"The kids now know our morning connection time is sacred - they call it 'Mom and Dad's Power-Up.' Funny! They've even started rating our family systems on a scale of 1-10. Last week our 8-year-old suggested an 'optimization' to bedtime routine. We're not just building our relationship; we're teaching them how to engineer their own future relationships."*

Next, we start Part 2 – ENGINEER. In **Chapter Five**, *The Relationship BUILD Framework*, you'll draft your personal plan for relationship growth based on your metrics from Part 1 - DECODE.

Remember: you already have the engineering mindset. Now let's apply it to what matters most!

PART II

ENGINEER

5

THE RELATIONSHIP BUILD FRAMEWORK - YOUR BLUEPRINT FOR SUCCESS

Sow a thought and you reap an action; sow an act and you reap a habit; sow a habit and you reap a character; sow a character and you reap a destiny

— RALPH WALDO EMERSON

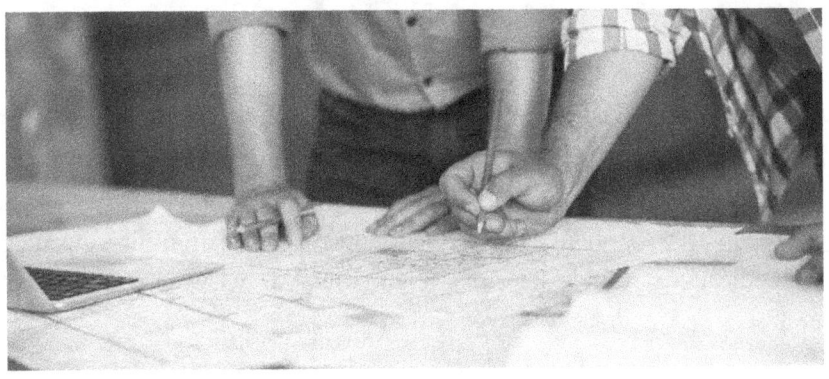

Real Life Scenario: The Kitchen Table Crisis in Kuala Lumpur

"It all came to a head during dinner," Elena explained, her hand clasping Wei's at their kitchen table. She worked as a school psychologist, while Wei was in water management. *"We were trying to arrange care for his mom who's battling cancer in Singapore, manage our daughter's cyberbullying problem at school, and figure out how to tell our youngest about the upcoming mortgage increase. Then the news showed war footage, triggering Wei's pandemic anxiety..."*

Wei shared, *"That's when our 12-year-old looked up from her plate and said, 'You guys don't laugh together anymore.' It wasn't just about us - but our whole family's emotional system."*

Such Stressed and Busy High-Performance Couples Often Ask Questions Like:

- How can we renew our couple connection in a way that works for our family?
- What kind of simple and effective recipe can we follow to rebuild our connection?

Overview

Every successful engineering project requires a precise blueprint – a systematic approach that guides implementation while allowing for strategic adjustments. The BUILD Framework provides exactly that: a comprehensive system for transforming your relationship through methodical, measurable steps that align with your achievement-oriented mindset.

This framework isn't about forcing rigid structures onto your relationship but creating a flexible architecture that supports natural connection while maintaining the efficiency you value. Just as you'd approach any complex project, the BUILD Framework breaks down relationship enhancement into clear, manageable phases that build upon each other systematically.

Through this engineering-inspired approach, you'll learn to:

- Structure relationship improvement as a series of achievable steps
- Establish clear metrics for tracking progress at each stage
- Design feedback loops for continuous optimization
- Develop sustainable systems for long-term connection

The BUILD Framework converts relationship renewal from an overwhelming challenge into a series of strategic implementations, each designed to create measurable improvements while respecting the constraints of your high-performance lifestyle.

EXPLAINING THE FIVE PHASES OF B.U.I.L.D FOR ENGINEERING UNBREAKABLE LOVE

As summarized earlier, **the Relationship BUILD Framework** is comprised of five phases: Base; Understand; Implement; Leverage; and Deepen. Each phase serves as a critical component in constructing unbreakable love. **BASE helps you start with solid metrics** on which you can plan goals and progress tracking systems for your relationship, to confidently increase connection.

The **UNDERSTAND phase** helps you analyze your daily interactions, map connection opportunities and understand each other's triggers. This enables you to plan strategic connection at times and in ways that give you the best results. You'll start *Morning Connection* rituals in Week One.

The **IMPLEMENT phase** assists you to build more love habits to reinforce your connection on a daily basis. *Midday Check-ins* start between Day 8-14, normalizing them in your routine and monitoring your connection levels, making your relationship more dynamic and hardier.

The **LEVERAGE phase** gets you capitalizing on your relationship strengths, refining patterns that work well and building on your successes to springboard further growth. Leverage incorporates *Evening Bonding* protocols between Day 15-21 to make your habits sustainable long-term.

The **DEEPEN phase** strengthens the architecture of your connection to establish lasting routines. Maintaining your couple engineering system is key. Further skill sharpening occurs during Day 22-28 with Part 3 – FORTIFY, advancing your love habits to the next level.

Your 28-Day Transformation Roadmap

Week 1: Getting Started

- Day 1-3: Assessment
- Day 4-7: Goal setting
- Action focus: Morning rituals

Week 2: Establishing Habits

- Day 8-14: Practice recording
- Implementation focus: Daytime connection
- Family rhythm integration

Week 3: Optimizing Connection

- Day 15-21: System optimization
- Strategic refinement: Evening habits
- Family adaptation support

Week 4: Consolidation and Celebration

- Day 22-28: Success amplification
- Sustainable integration: Routine set
- Longterm connection enhancement

Applying Kolb's Experiential Learning Cycle to Your Couple Connection

This well-known theory argues that we can learn from our daily experiences and treats reflection as an integral part of such learning. According to Kolb (1984), the process of learning follows a pattern or cycle consisting of four stages, one of which Kolb refers to as 'reflective observation.' Engineering unbreakable love is supported best by adopting an experiential learning approach as a couple. The stages are illustrated and summarised below.

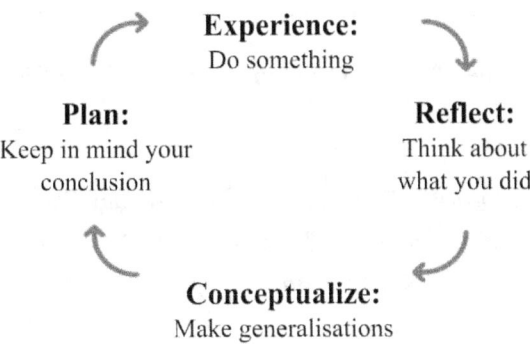

SETTING MEASURABLE OUTCOMES AND IMPLEMENTATION STRATEGIES

In a fast-paced world where each moment counts, setting measurable goals for your relationship can turn vague hopes into tangible achievements. Applying strategies from tech and business settings, can ensure your relationship progress is both visible and achievable.

To start with, be specific in setting relationship goals, like the S.M.A.R.T.A.R. criteria - Specific, Measurable, Attainable, Relevant, Time-bound, Agreed-on and Reviewed. Structured goal setting that is agreed-upon boosts the likelihood of achievement. By specifying timeframes and measuring progress, you create urgency and focus that motivates you both to keep going.

To further support attainment of measurable goals, consider how you leverage technology to track and monitor progress. Digital tools like shared calendars or goal-tracking apps, can provide reminders and facilitate accountability. *Documenting your goals and progress in our Relationship Vitality Dashboard will give you visible records of your efforts.* These tools can help you share insights and feedback, fostering transparency and enhancing communication.

Your Action Steps:

Discuss your metrics then plan specific connection goals to achieve by Day 7.

For example, higher **Baseline Connection** stats, quality **KCIs** or improved **6MC** use.

> # What will be better by Day 14, for example - **Midday Check-Ins?**
> # How about aiming for higher **TIC** scores out of 10, by Day 21?
> # What is your couple **Relationship Vitality** goal - out of 10 - by Day 28?
> # What actionable strategies are you going to use to achieve these goals?

Implementation strategies benefit from mutual support and accountability, just as successful firms rely on collaborative teamwork. Your relationship will thrive when you warmly encourage each other's efforts. A simple system like daily check-ins on shared goals can reinforce your dedication to the process and ensure your efforts are aligned. This prepares you for the next phase, where you will leverage your strengths to build on the progress you have made.

The Reality of Modern Love within Elena and Wei's Weekly Lifecycle:

- Monday: Virtual check-in with Wei's mom's oncologist in Singapore
- Tuesday: Daughter's therapy for cyberbullying

- Wednesday: Elena's sister needs support through divorce
- Thursday: Community food bank volunteering
- Friday: Family nature walk - their 'sanity reset'
- Weekend: Balancing temple visits with kids' sports

THE POWER OF LOVE HABITS IN CONNECTING WITH NATURE

Elena and Wei's discovery: *"Our Saturday morning park walks became sacred. Something about being in nature helps us process everything - from mom's cancer updates to mortgage stress. Our kids open up more, we breathe easier, and problems feel more manageable."*

Key Takeaway 5: A structured framework provides clear direction for relationship renewal while honoring life's complexities.

CLOSING REFLECTION AND SUCCESS STORY

Elena and Wei's update two months on: *"We still have all the same challenges - mom's cancer, kid's school stress, mortgage payments. But now we have connection habits to handle them together. Last week, during our park walk, we found ourselves laughing at a family joke while organizing mom's treatment program. That's when we knew - we'd moved forward."*

In Chapter Six, *BASE - Foundation Setting*, we help you clarify the connection times and methods you want to use for your couple goals, as you start on the 28-Day Roadmap.

6

BASE - FOUNDATION SETTING

Whoever acts on these words is like the wise person who built their house on the rock. The rains came down, the streams rose, and the winds blew and beat against that house; yet it did not fall because it had its foundations on the rock

— JESUS CHRIST

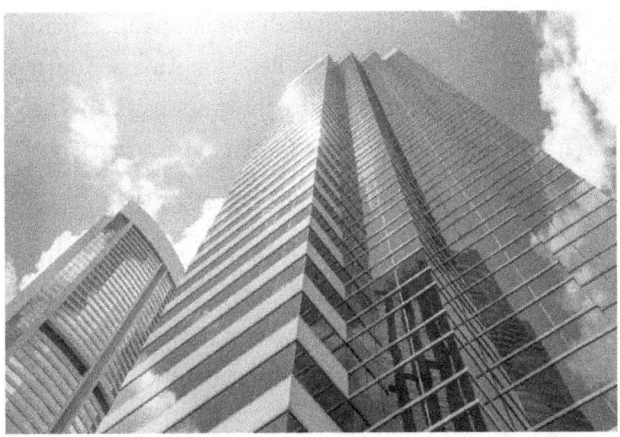

Real Life Scenario: Electric Power Loss in South Africa

The darkness was a gift, Thabo realized, as another night of power cuts left their Johannesburg home in shadows. Thabo's work in IT meant he knew how much business depends on virtual connection, just as his wife Amara's financial acumen was integral to her CFO role in their tech startup, and to all aspects of their lives. Now their three school-aged children had finally settled, their phones glowing faintly under pillows despite *"no devices after dinner."* He found Amara on their balcony, her silhouette outlined against the city's patchy lights, with some neighborhoods bright while others waited in darkness for their power to return.

"Remember the first-time electricity stopped after moving here?" she asked as he joined her. *"I was still learning to navigate South Africa, missing Lagos terribly, and you taught me to see these blackouts as forced moments of pause. We were then able to reflect together on what was working in our new life here and what would help us feel connected as a couple and family."*

He slipped his hand into hers, remembering that first year - her struggling to blend Nigerian traditions with their new life, his father's dementia diagnosis, the endless demands of their business. *"Now look at us,"* he smiled. *"We've built our own power cut reflection ritual."*

Their ritual had evolved organically. When the power died, phones would be gathered in the 'technology tomb,' (their youngest's dramatic name for the kitchen drawer). Candles would be lit with intention rather than frustration. Stories would flow first - Nigerian folktales from Amara, Zulu legends from their children's school, dreams of future innovations from Thabo, and as a result - meaningful couple talk occurred when the kids had gone back to bed.

The link between electricity supply pausing and your relationship status might be noticing your need to slow down and reflect when you two feel disconnected. *It might not be prompted by external events like electricity blackouts, but what is it that you notice when you realize your couple connection is suffering?* This is why taking your ***Connection Baseline*** and doing morning ***6-Minute Connect*** practices are key. Then note your metrics and experiences so you can ask *"What re-connection methods do we need most, right now? And how shall we achieve that?"*

High-Performance Couples Seeking Stronger Connection Ask Questions Like:

- What specific steps can we take to create and measure our connection baselines?
- What short-term goals will be realistic for us to achieve improved connection soon?

Overview

Every masterful engineering project starts with solid foundations. Just as you wouldn't construct a building without first analyzing the soil and establishing proper footings, your relationship renewal requires careful baseline assessment and clear metrics.

Base-setting isn't just about gathering data, it's about creating the infrastructure that supports lasting change. For high-achievers who understand the value of proper groundwork, this phase provides the steps needed to track and validate relationship progress. Creating clear baselines and measurement systems will help you turn intuitive couple dynamics into trackable metrics.

Through systematic foundation setting, you'll:

- Create precise measurements for relationship vitality
- Establish clear benchmarks for progress tracking
- Design efficient monitoring systems in your Dashboard
- Build accountability that drives consistent improvement

This foundational phase ensures your future love engineering efforts are built on solid metrics to inform you, goals to guide your progress and tracking to validate your success.

ASSESSMENT TOOLS AND METRICS

Like Thabo and Amara, it pays to slow down and think carefully about what works and what else would help? This is an act of love – to be the archaeologists, examining your foundations. To set the base for a thriving partnership, you must make an accurate assessment to clarify your connection levels, then identify how to intentionally enhance these.

Understanding your relationship through assessment tools and metrics allows you to approach your partnership with the same analytical precision you apply in your professional life.

Reflection and Action Questions:

Did you self-assess in our introduction to **Connection Baselines** *in Chapter One?*

Whether you have or not yet, I invite you to do the exercise below to find *what connection methods help most and what you two need more of*. If you did the exercises and noted your metrics in your **Relationship Vitality Dashboard**, *what are your most pressing couple needs?*

For example, if you noticed in your **Connection Baseline** that you need more focused attention, emotional sharing, meaningful touch or playfulness, *which one is most urgent to you? Which one does your partner need?* Look back at your metrics. *What did you find?* If you still need to, do those now and record your findings on the Chart, to see what is most important to you both.

Remember to use the **Relationship Vitality Dashboard** at the end of Chapter 3 to capture the key metrics and insights from your Relationship Assessments. This Dashboard is designed as a 'go to tool' for you to see where you are at and what you need to succeed.

GOAL ALIGNMENT STRATEGIES

In couple relating, aligned goals are key to building an enjoyable and enduring partnership.

Now, back to considering your most urgent needs found by doing your **Connection Baseline.** *Let's say it was emotional sharing that she needs more of and more meaningful touch for him. Ok – how much more is realistic to practice giving each other in the next 7 Days?*

Your answers will clarify these goals and then you just add a few details to make your goals SMARTAR. Specific, Measurable, Attainable, Relevant, Time-bound, Agreed-on and Reviewed.

 # How many times per day will you plan to give emotional sharing of your thoughts and feelings?

 # And if you plan to give more meaningful affectionate touches – how many each day?

 # What amount do you both plan to be giving by Day 7?

At this stage, I am inviting you to join me on a 28-Day process, *therefore please choose how many of these connections you want to be making by Day 7 and 14? Then by Day 21 and 28?*

In addition to setting joint goals, it is essential to plan regular check-ins. *When will you do that?* These provide times to discuss your progress, address challenges, and adjust your approaches.

Progress Tracking Systems

In dynamic high-performance relationships, just setting goals is not enough; tracking progress is crucial to ensure that these goals translate into meaningful outcomes. That is why I designed the **Relationship Dashboard** charts for you to use throughout reading this book and beyond.

Further, why not look strategically into your couple future and think about how you will maintain conscious intentional love habits into the next 3-12 months? Or 12-24 months?

COUPLE CONNECTION METHODS - THE TECHNOLOGY OF TOUCH

Back in Johannesburg, Thabo and Amara were learning how to engineer intimacy during another power cut, as Amara shared her mother's teachings about touch languages.

"In our village," she said, signing on Thabo's palm, *"every touch was a word, every gesture a sentence. We didn't need electricity to communicate love."* They began developing their own touch vocabulary. A finger traced on a wrist during morning rush meant *"I see you."* A hand on the shoulder while passing said, *"I support you."* Three quick squeezes translated to *"I love you."*

CLOSING REFLECTION AND SUCCESS STORY: RECORDING YOUR COUPLE CONNECTION QUALITY ACROSS YOUR 28-DAY ROADMAP

As power resumed in Johannesburg, Thabo and Amara's house hummed back to life. Their children emerged from their blanket forts, phones reactivated, screens glowed. But something had shifted during those dark hours.

"Maybe," Amara mused, watching their youngest show Thabo a drawing made by candlelight, *"we needed these forced pauses to build our real power system."* Thabo nodded agreement. They had engineered something precious in the darkness - a foundation that didn't depend on external power but generated its own light.

Key Takeaway 6: Establishing clear baseline metrics enables targeted improvement.

Remember: Strong couple connection and metrics don't stop life's crises happening, but they provide the supportive foundation to face the storms of life and stay solid together. Take time throughout the book to record your metrics below on your *28-Day Roadmap Progress Chart.*

In Chapter Seven, *UNDERSTAND - Connection Mapping,* we help you find times to connect.

Your 28-Day Transformation Roadmap:

Week 1: Getting Started

- Day 1-3: Assessment ✅
- Day 4-7: Goal setting ✅
- Action focus: Morning rituals ✅

Week 2: Establishing Habits

- Day 8-14: Practice recording
- Implementation focus: Daytime connection
- Family rhythm integration

Week 3: Optimizing Connection

- Day 15-21: System optimization
- Strategic refinement: Evening habits
- Family adaptation support

Week 4: Consolidation and Celebration

- Day 22-28: Success amplification
- Sustainable integration: Routine set
- Longterm connection enhancement

98 | BASE - FOUNDATION SETTING

Recording Your Couple Connection Quality Across Your 28-Day Roadmap

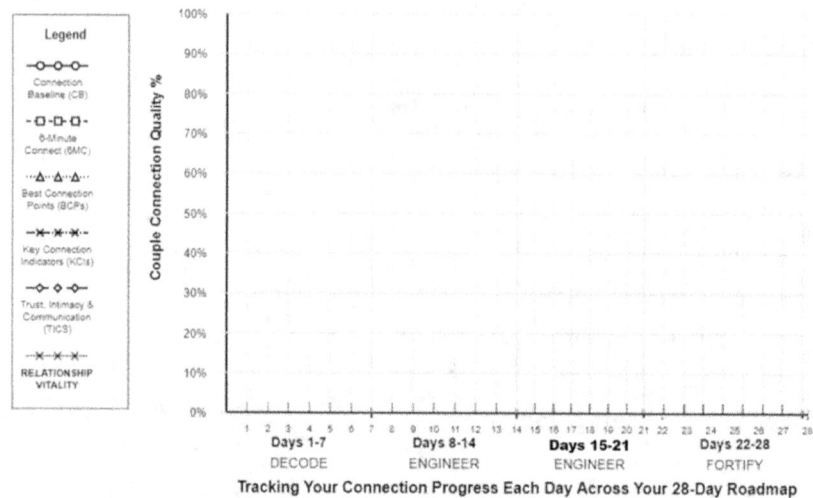

Tracking Your Connection Progress Each Day Across Your 28-Day Roadmap

See Michael and Sarah's real life 28-Day Roadmap from Chapter One below. They scored each metric line with its symbols - in pencil, pen, crayon and black markers. Yes, its messy, but it was effective! Take heart, their six metrics all started out between 30-50% at Day 1 and were up to 50-70% by Day 28, thanks to their dogged determination to build connection, 'little and often' using their tailored love habits. The grey bands depict their initial goals, which they achieved!

Michael and Sarah's Couple Connection Quality Across Their 28-Day Roadmap

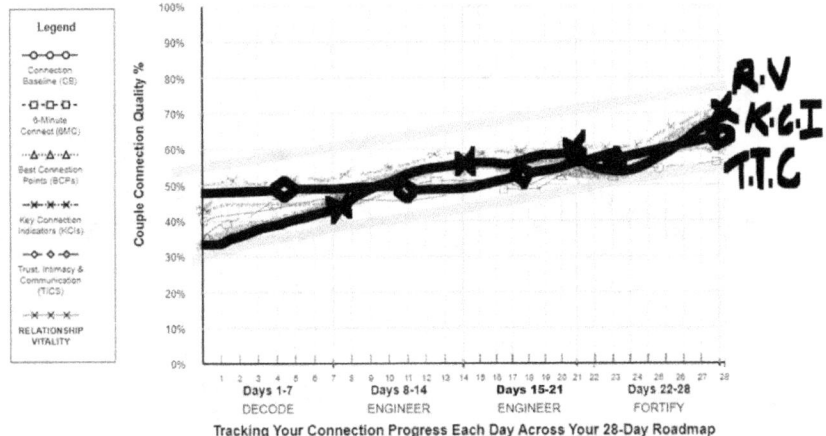

Tracking Your Connection Progress Each Day Across Your 28-Day Roadmap

7

UNDERSTAND - CONNECTION MAPPING

The opportunity of a lifetime must be seized during the lifetime of the opportunity

— LEONARD RAVENHILL

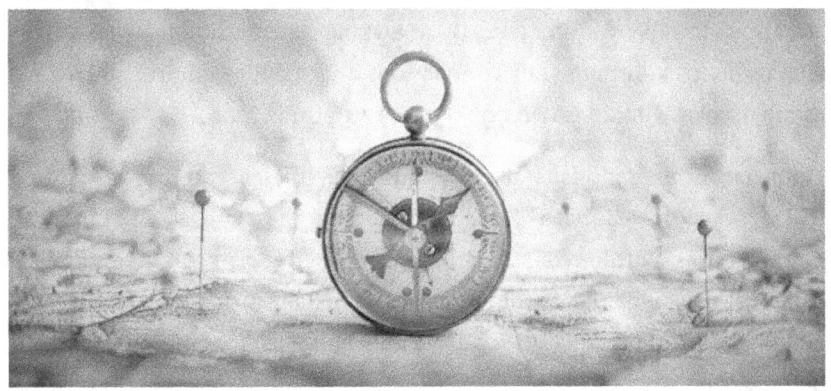

Real Life Scenario: The Language of Memory in Osaka

Yuki, a clothing textiles engineer whispered, *"It's not just cloth,"* spreading her nana's wedding kimono carefully across their Osaka apartment floor. Cherry blossom petals drifted past their window as Hamish knelt beside his pregnant wife, learning to read the fabric's story.

"Each pattern speaks," Yuki continued, tracing a golden thread. *"See how these waves weave into mountains? Like our story, your Scottish highlands meeting my ocean heritage."* Hamish's aerospace engineering mind began to see new kinds of patterns in the silk before them.

High-Performance Couples Seeking to Map Connection Times Ask Questions Like:

- What are the most critical connection points in our day?
- How do we identify genuine connection opportunities?
- What triggers our disconnection patterns?
- How do we create new patterns without disrupting our routine?

Overview

Relationships, like all complex systems, follow discernible patterns, and reward is found by systematically analyzing and optimizing these. This chapter helps you map your connections and manage emotional triggers as precisely as you do professional process optimization.

Connection mapping isn't about imposing artificial structure on natural interactions. Instead, it's about recognizing the natural rhythms and opportunities within your existing routines. By using your analytical skills within your relationship dynamics, you can turn sudden emotional responses into predictable, manageable patterns to be optimized for better connection.

Through strategic connection mapping, you'll learn to:

- Identify the best connection opportunities in your daily schedule
- Recognize emotional trigger patterns and response cycles
- Map optimal connection points within current time usage
- Create systematic approaches to emotional awareness

Understanding these patterns transforms relationship enhancement from guesswork into a precise science, allowing you to engineer connection points that work in your busy lifestyle.

DAILY INTERACTION ANALYSIS - UNDERSTANDING CONNECTION MAPPING

In the whirlwind of life, where the demands of career, family, and personal growth intersect, understanding connection opportunities is key. Consider Yuki and Hamish, whose days are filled with emails, meetings, and product development. Yet, amidst this busyness, they noticed a growing distance in their relationship. They long for the kind of enjoyment together that they find in their work roles. Enter the concept of connection mapping, to find times to connect better, much like learning the coding of a complex program.

Opportunity Mapping

To understand what times you might best connect with each other, examine the daily routines you share with your partner. Consider the habitual patterns that shape your days, from morning rituals to evening wind-downs. *Within these routines lie numerous opportunities for connection, often hidden in plain sight.* For instance, the commute to work can be seen as a mundane necessity or intentionally turned into a time of shared reflection or planning.

Similarly, preparing meals together can evolve from a chore into a shared creative endeavor, fostering teamwork and communication. *By consciously* seeking these opportunities, you can choose moments in your routine to reinforce your partnership and contribute to its vitality.

Did you try this in our earlier **Connection Point Mapping** with Richard and Lisa in Chapter Two? If not, I suggest you flick back there and review their example opportunities for connecting. If you have not done it yet, do the exercise below to find when is best for you to connect: transition times; cross-over moments; previously missed chances; or new ways you can connect.

Exercise: Connection Point Mapping to Discover Your Best Connection Points (10mins)

1. List your daily transition points
2. Identify existing touch points
3. Note current missed opportunities
4. Mark potential new connection moments

Your Implementation Plan: Mapping and Using BCPs for Connection and Learning

Today:

- Complete *Connection Point Mapping*
    - Identify three potential Best Connection Points (BCPs)
    - Plan to discuss action steps e.g 'Use *6MC* Daily'

This Week:

- Choose one BCP to implement
    - Design specific protocol
    - Use the recording Chart

This Fortnight:

- Add two more BCPs
  - Refine timing and approach
  - Document impact and adjustment

Recording a Trial Week of Utilizing BCPs for Connection and Learning:

Daily Number of Successful BCPs	Average Quality of Each BCP Connection	Impact on Emotional State of Both Partners	Effect on Relationship Satisfaction Reported
Monday =			
Tuesday =			
Wednesday =			
Thursday =			
Friday =			
Saturday =			
Sunday =			
Average = /Day	Quality =		

Opportunity mapping takes a shift in perception, to view challenges as potential catalysts for connection. For example, the demands of parenting, elderly care, or maintaining a household are responsibilities that can feel overwhelming. *Instead of viewing these tasks as burdens, try reframing them as shared projects to practice collaboration and mutual support.*

TRIGGER IDENTIFICATION

If you want to preserve relationships, then you must learn to respond *instead of* reacting *to fear and pain. You can* react *without thinking but you cannot* respond *without training your mind to think, your will to choose, and your body to obey*

— DANNY SILK

Understanding the triggers that disconnect you by influencing your emotional responses is a pivotal step in sustaining a healthy relationship. These triggers from past experiences or early relationships can evoke strong emotions of inadequacy, rejection, or abandonment, affecting how you react to your partner during conflicts or stress. Recognizing and understanding these triggers enables you to handle them with greater empathy and recover connection more quickly.

Reflection Questions:

Recall moments in your interactions where you felt an out of proportion emotional response – either over or under-reacting, whether it was anger, sadness, or anxiety. What circumstances led to these reactions? Identify any recurring patterns or themes. What actions bring you calm and comfort - returning your body and nervous system to safety?

The best thing you can do is let your partner know in advance how to help in those moments, like preparing sandbags before the emotional floods hit. If you need further assistance, you could try Matt Brown's *InnerBoy* App for blokes and get therapeutic help as required.

Couple Case Study: The Garden's Teaching

Dawn in Osaka found Yuki and Hamish by their container garden. *"The moss,"* Yuki explained, *"only grows when we respect its patterns. Too much water, it drowns. Too little, it withers."*

Over time, they would go on to learn how to read each other like they read their garden. Hamish needed physical movement when processing emotions, like his Scottish ancestors who paced heather-covered hills. Yuki's quiet spells did not mean withdrawal but deep contemplation, like the still surface of a temple pond. These patterns informed when and how to connect best.

COUPLE STORIES AND CLOSING REFLECTIONS

Example - When Patterns Break

Late one night in their Osaka home, Hamish found Yuki crying over their broken tea bowl. *"It was my dear nana's,"* Yuki explained, holding the pieces. But then she smiled through her tears, tracing the gold seams where it had been repaired years before.

"Kintsugi," she explained to Hamish. *"The art of making broken things beautiful."* They sat on their kitchen floor, seeing how the gold lines created new patterns, telling stories of breaking and healing. *"Maybe,"* Hamish said, given their arguments lately, *"Our relationship patterns are like this too. When they break, we can make something stronger in the mending."*

Second Example – How Connection Happened

As another night of power cuts settled over Johannesburg, Thabo and Amara sat with their connection map spread before them - not a chart or diagram, but a collection of stories, moments, and patterns they'd noticed over months of paying attention.

"Look," Amara pointed out, *"how our best conversations happen in darkness. How the children always sleep better when we sing your mother's lullabies. How your best coding happens after our morning prayer time."*

Thabo added his own observations - the way Amara's voice changed when she needed support but couldn't ask directly. How their youngest always sensed tension and cleared it with sudden laughter. The patterns of their love across blackouts and bright times. *"We're not just mapping connection,"* he realized. *"We're mapping home."*

Key Takeaway 7: Understanding patterns reveals natural connection opportunities.

Remember: Around the world, couples are discovering the patterns of their shared lives. Like gardeners reading seasons, mapping connection with each other, one pattern at a time.

In Chapter Eight, *IMPLEMENT - Strategic Connection Points*, you will plan and practice connection at the times in your days that you have mapped out as being most conducive.

8

IMPLEMENT - STRATEGIC CONNECTION POINTS

A little here, a little there; like the steady dripping of water, small acts done consistently over time can carve great canyons

— UNKNOWN

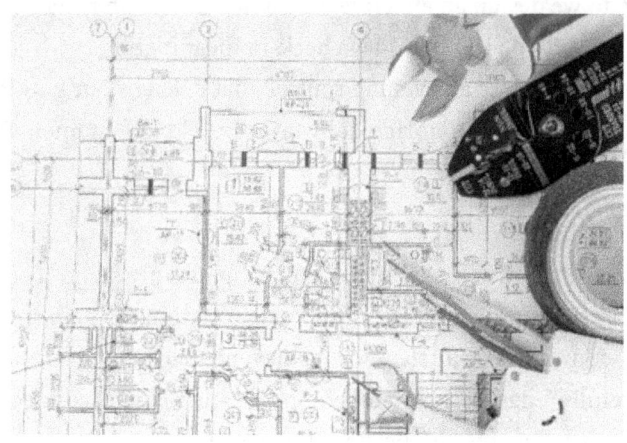

110 | IMPLEMENT - STRATEGIC CONNECTION POINTS

Real Life Scenario: Sacred Time in Switzerland

The early morning fog wrapped around the hills of Zurich as Omar slipped out of bed, careful not to wake his sleeping wife Freda. In the kitchen, he quietly moved through their ritual - grinding coffee beans from the roaster where they'd had their first date, warming milk in the pan Freda's mother insisted they take from Berlin. Omar knew Freda loved nothing more than to wake up to the smell of coffee made and brought to her in bed, as part of their morning connect.

Omar's device flashed with emails from his landscape architecture students, but this calm moment - this was theirs. Omar watched the steam rise from two cups, remembering how his late grandmother in Ankara, Türkiye had run her own café. He poignantly imagined her face and voice, *"she would be so proud to see me loving Freda this way by bringing her morning coffee,"* he mused. Omar smiled with love and pride, reflecting on his family's closeness and Freda's success in the finance sector. It was time to take the fresh brew to his waking wife.

High-Performance Couples Crafting Intentional Love Habits Often Ask:

- How do we design an effective morning connection ritual?
- What exactly makes a midday check-in meaningful?
- How do we create an evening routine that deepens our bond?
- What could turn our boring daily tasks into loving moments?

Overview

Implementation is where engineering principles truly shine. This chapter turns theoretical understanding into practical action through strategically designed connection rituals. For achievement-oriented professionals, these carefully engineered touchpoints create reliable connection that improve rather than disrupt peak performance.

The key to sustainable relationship growth lies not in grand gestures but in precisely engineered micro-moments. By designing strategic connection points throughout your day, you create a systematic approach to intimacy that aligns with your lifestyle. Each interaction becomes an opportunity for intentional connection.

Your implementation strategies will enable you to:

- Transform daily transitions into connection opportunities
- Create efficient protocols for meaningful interaction
- Design scalable systems for consistent intimacy
- Build reliable methods for emotional engagement

Strategic implementation ensures that every connection point serves a specific purpose in strengthening your relationship architecture.

For many couples, the morning sets the tone for the day ahead, offering an opportunity to connect before the world demands your attention. Imagine starting each day with a ritual designed to bring you closer, anchoring your relationship in the calm before the chaos. This chapter explores the art of morning ritual design and midday check-ins, so both can be well implemented to deepen your bond and foster unity that lasts through the day.

MORNING RITUAL DESIGN

Morning rituals mean more than just rising and starting the day - they are deliberate practices including mindfulness, gratitude, and shared experiences to boost your relationship. Research has shown that couples engaging in consistent, meaningful rituals report higher levels of satisfaction and closeness, as these habits strengthen their bond. The morning, with its fresh start and promise of possibility, is an ideal time to make these rituals part of your routine.

Reflection Questions:

If you tried the 3-Day Challenge earlier, how did your 6-Minute Connect in the mornings go? Did you try using the 6MC at any other connection points in your day?

In crafting your morning rituals to suit you, consider what activities help you to engage. I remind you of the *6-Minute Connect* ideas provided earlier. Firstly, eye contact over a cuppa, sharing a full embrace and focusing on each other – being fully present in the moment. Second, sharing one hope for the day, or concern and offering a caring response can bond you deeply. Thirdly, giving a short thank you, intention to be in touch later and closing with a hug or physical touch. These short exchanges can build appreciation and warmth between you, which aligns with principles from the Gottman Method, of daily kindness being essential for sustaining love.

Your Action Steps: Trial Your 6-Minute Connect – Record Notes Here Afterward:

Components to Practice	Quality and Impact	Relationship Satisfaction
First 2 Minutes: Present Moment	E.g Ok. Good. Helped	Low. Ok. Good. High. Great
Make eye contact over cuppa		
Share a full embrace		
Focus together - phones away		
2 Minutes: Emotional Check-In		
Share one hope for the day		
Express a concern or vulnerability		
Offer supporting acknowledgment		
2 Minutes: Thankful & Intention		
Express gratitude for recent thing		
Set connection intention for today		
Meaningful physical contact		
Overall – How was Your '6-Minute	Morning Connect?'	You Feel?

For couples who thrive on physical activity, joint exercise in your mornings provide both bodily and emotional benefits. Whether a brisk walk, yoga session, or quick workout, such activity together promotes health and vitality with shared accomplishment. The endorphins released during exercise can charge you with positivity, energizing your interactions.

Keeping your morning connection ritual effective means shaping it dynamically to respond to your changing needs. Regularly assess what parts resonate with you both and adjust your ritual to ensure it stays fulfilling, not monotonous or obligatory. You may want to try out seasonal variations or explore new activities to keep it fresh and engaging.

MIDDAY CHECK-IN OPTIMIZATION

During demanding days, finding moments to reconnect with your partner can be tricky. Yet, it is precisely at these times that a brief, intentional check-in can be a refreshing lifeline. *To keep it simple and achievable, these* **Midday Check-ins** *can just be an adapted version of your morning* **6MC**. You can still connect emotionally without being physically close, as in the example below.

Midday Check-ins *are not interruptions; they are strategic touchpoints designed to maintain emotional closeness, ensuring both partners feel valued. Think of them like the relational equivalent of a software update - brief, efficient, and vital for optimal functioning.*

As you plough through the myriad tasks in your role, a **Midday Check-in** offers a pause to refresh your emotional connection. *These may include gratitude for efforts made at home, a quick update from the morning, or asking about each other's well-being.* Responding positively like this to daily bids for attention can significantly bolster trust and emotional intimacy.

To optimize these check-ins, use the mode of communication that suits your needs. For some, a quick phone call may suffice, offering the comfort of hearing your partner's voice. Alternatively, a brief text or digital note might suit best when schedules are tight. The medium matters less than the intention - what counts is that they feel like your top priority. This bonding assures both individuals that they are thought of and valued, like Omar and Freda did in the example below.

Your Midday Check-In Example (Adapted 6MC). Record Your Trial Notes Here:

TWO SHORT CONNECTION STEPS	Quality and Impact	Relationship Satisfaction
Thankful Moment & Update	*E.g Ok. Good. Helped*	*E.g Ok. Good. High. Great*
Express gratitude for recent action		
Ask / say how morning tasks went		
Emotional Validate & Check-In		
Validate one feeling shared above		
Offer support and hope to connect		
Overall: How was Your 'Midday	**Connect?'**	**You Feel?**

Incorporating a structured element into your *Midday Check-in* can enhance its effectiveness, and this may suit using a shared digital tool or app if you are not already. While consistency is important, flexibility remains key. Life has a way of disrupting even the best-laid plans, and there will be days when a check-in may need to be delayed. When needed, a quick acknowledgment of the day's demands, with a promise to reconnect later, can suffice.

TWO SHORT CONNECTION STEPS	Quality and Impact	Relationship Satisfaction
Thankful Moment & Update	*E.g Ok. Good. Helped*	*E.g Ok. Good. High. Great*
Express gratitude for recent action	Good. Felt appreciated	Good
Ask / say how morning tasks went	Ok. Nice to be asked	Good
Emotional Validate & Check-In		
Validate one feeling shared above	Good, helped feel seen	High
Offer support and hope to connect	Great. Keen on hug tonight	Great, feel closer as result
Overall: How was Your 'Midday	**Connect?'** *Really helpful*	**You Feel?** *Glad and loved*

*All this was achieved in a five-minute video call that switched to phone, due to signal lapse.

EVENING BONDING HABITS

As the day ends and energy wanes, the evening is a chance to reconnect. While this is true, *remember - introverts need time alone to recharge their batteries.* And, if you have children, their needs will be central at night, as with Marcus and Maya in Chapter Four. Your evenings can be tailored around what suits your energies, families and household needs.

To keep things easy, *you could use a night version of your* **6MC** *ritual here.* When designing evening bonding habits, use shared experiences that increase closeness and relaxation. For example, whether you garden, do sudoku, watch TV, take walks, listen to music, play darts or table tennis, such activities can provide a comforting sense of companionable togetherness.

The power of touch cannot be overstated. Physical closeness, whether hugs, holding hands, or a gentle massage, has been shown to release oxytocin, a hormone that promotes feelings of trust and security. These simple acts of physical connection can help partners decompress and transition from the stresses of the day to a more relaxed, intimate state.

Creating an environment conducive to relaxation helps evening bonding rituals. Use of soft lighting, calming music, or aromatic scents that promote tranquility, can create an inviting and soothing space. By crafting your environment this way, you signal to your partner that this time is sacred, dedicated to the nurturing of your relationship.

Conversation is a part of the glue in your evening bonding, as you reflect on the day's events, share thoughts and feelings, and discuss plans for the future. By focusing on positive words and affirmations, you reinforce the emotional warmth and acceptance in your partnership.

Action Step:

With your morning, noon and night connection rituals in mind, now let's reassess your *KCIs*.

Review Your Connection KCIs. Record Your Metrics and Experiences Here:

THREE TYPES OF CONNECTION	Quantity and Quality	Relationship Satisfaction
Physical Connection Metrics	E.g 1-2. Ok. Good. Helped	Low. Good. High. Great
Daily affectionate touches		
Non-sexual physical affection		
Sleep proximity patterns		
Sexually intimate moments		
Emotional Connection Metrics		
Deep conversations initiated		
Vulnerable shares exchanged		
Supportive moments offered		
Joint parenting wins		
Mental Connection Metrics		
Shared decisions made		
Problems solved together		
Future plans discussed		
Parenting strategies aligned		
Overall: How is Your Three-Fold	Connection?	You Feel?

CLOSING REFLECTION AND SUCCESS STORY

The Power of Daily Love Habits

Strong connection can be built by applying the wisdom of 'little and often,' as Freda reflected. *"It is so lovely to be cared for first thing in my day when Omar brings me coffee and we sit quietly drinking it together. Then when he contacts me at work for our midday check-in, that feeling deepens, which helps me look forward to cuddling with him at home in the evenings."*

Key Takeaway 8: Strategic implementation creates sustainable connection habits.

Remember: Small acts of love done often accumulate to build deep bonds that last.

In Chapter Nine, *LEVERAGE - System Optimization*, we will optimize the approaches you have found successful to maximize your relationship growth.

Your 28-Day Transformation Roadmap:

Week 1: Getting Started

- Day 1-3: Assessment ✅
- Day 4-7: Goal setting ✅
- Action focus: Morning rituals ✅

Week 2: Establishing Habits

- Day 8-14: Practice recording ✅
- Implementation focus: Daytime connection ✅
- Family rhythm integration

Week 3: Optimizing Connection

- Day 15-21: System optimization
- Strategic refinement: Evening habits
- Family adaptation support

Week 4: Consolidation and Celebration

- Day 22-28: Success amplification
- Sustainable integration: Routine set
- Longterm connection enhancement

9

LEVERAGE - SYSTEM OPTIMIZATION

Success is the sum of small efforts, repeated day in and day out

— ROBERT COLLIER

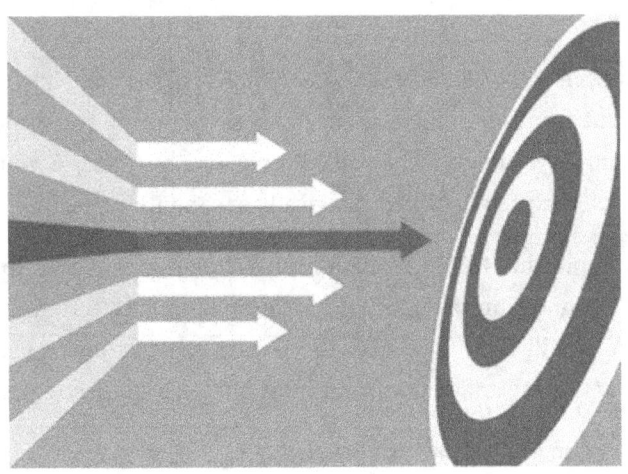

Real Life Scenario: The Pattern Perfectors in Chile

Dawn in Santiago found Zach, a senior medical officer, adjusting their 'Connection Calendar,' in light of his wife Ava's paediatric specialist roster. He wasn't adding new moments but optimizing those they'd found. *"It's like fine-tuning code,"* Zach explained to Ava over their morning chai. *"We know these connection points work. Now let's make them work better."*

Zach, fresh from his hospital shift, understood optimization intuitively. *"Like in surgery - once you master the basic procedure, you find ways to make it more efficient, more effective."*

High-Performance Couples Finding Love Habits Beneficial Tend to Ask:

- How do we maintain momentum once we see improvement?
- What adjustments will create even stronger connections?
- How do we prevent falling back into old patterns?
- What metrics show us how we're continuing to grow?

Overview

High-achievers know success comes not only from implementing systems, but from optimizing them for peak performance. System optimization improves relationships like it improves business, as you identify what works, analyze why and strategically expand its application.

Here we apply this to your relationship, showing you how to amplify successful connection patterns and scale their impact across your partnership. You will then maximize the return on your emotional investment by replicating and scaling your most effective connection practices.

Through systematic optimization, you'll:

- Identify and analyze your best connection moments

- Scale successful practices across different contexts
- Create multiplication effects from proven strategies
- Build self-reinforcing cycles of positive interaction

Optimization turns random successes into reliable systems, fine-tuning your connection habits to ensure consistent relationship growth with maximum efficiency. This chapter helps you refine the patterns that form the backbone of your bond, to nurture it with precision and intent.

PATTERN REFINEMENT

Connection patterns, like routines, shape the dynamics of your relationship. They are the formed habits and ways that you interact with your partner daily, like *6MCs*. These patterns, when positive, create fulfilling resilient partnerships, but when negative and unchecked, lead to stagnation or conflict. The first step in refining these patterns is recognizing their presence.

By now, you will have observed what helps your connection with your partner and what serves to strengthen your trust, deepen intimacy and improve your communication. I hope you have celebrated some warmer emotional exchanges and effective problem-solving recently.

Refining patterns involves teamwork as partners, including open dialogue about how these patterns affect your relationship. This process requires vulnerability and willingness to explore uncomfortable truths, while also providing invitations to heal and grow. Working together to refine your patterns deepens empathy, where both partners feel valued and understood.

Reflection Questions:

In your process of pattern refinement, what couple habits engender more positive dynamics?

What external factors (e.g work, family or personal pressures) affect your relationship most?

For instance, if you notice a pattern of miscommunication during stressful times, use your **Midday Check-ins** to allow each other to share thoughts and feelings without judgment. This can address the immediate issue and strengthen your overall communication. Such intentional habits serve as anchors, stabilizing your relationship amid the ebb and flow of life's demands.

SUCCESS AMPLIFICATION

Amplifying connection success is just as vital in relationships as it is in business, where a well-executed product launch elevates a company's standing. Likewise, celebrating and building on relational successes notably enhances your bond. Identifying moments of triumph – whether small connections or major changes – reinforces positive behavior and builds an expectation of more successful closeness in your relationship.

Recording your metrics is a great way to recognize and articulate these successes clearly, and value the efforts made to connect each day. Shining a light on these moments validates your contributions with appreciation and respect.

After this, the next step is to amplify their impact through deliberate reinforcement.

Reflection Questions:

What made a love habit most beneficial? Was it the words, touch, playfulness, emotional sharing, mutual support, gratitude or shared goal that helped you both the most?

By noticing these elements and their role in your successes, you can consciously replicate and enhance them in future. This is how you design feedback loops, so positive outcomes inform and shape your ongoing relationship. Then this cycle of success can become self-sustaining, strengthening the already robust foundation of your partnership.

The amplification of success also involves celebrating achievements in meaningful ways that show appreciation. Simple expressions of gratitude can make a big difference overall to your **Key Connection Indicators**. My wife and I do this daily, and our gratitude is flourishing.

Celebrating past connection successes sets the stage for future triumphs, growing a culture of progress and innovation between you. This helps you explore new experiences and opportunities for learning, which will further amplify your successes, ensuring that your relationship stays vibrant and resilient in the face of change.

STRATEGY SCALING

Scaling effective strategies in relationships echoes the principle in successful businesses, taking proven emotional engagement methods then expanding them to permeate every aspect of your shared life. This not only enhances the quality of your relationship but also ensures the connection remains robust and adaptable. Scaling relational strategies requires intentionality and foresight, like it does in business, when scaling a successful product demands careful planning and execution. It starts with asking yourselves, *"What worked well so far and what do we want more of? What parts of our current love habits shall we improve and measure?"*

Scaling strategies involve a thoughtful examination of your current lifestyle and commitments. The same principle of resource allocation that you use at work applies in your relationship, as you think about how to allocate your time, energy, and attention to amplify the impact of these successful connection strategies. It is about creating a daily and weekly rhythm that supports consistent engagement and connection, allowing your relationship to thrive.

Be aware that as your relationship and family stages change, you may need to adjust the ways you spend time together or redefine what connection looks like in your current phase of life.

Scaling strategies within your relationship requires knowing your metrics, especially your **KCIs**, setting SMARTAR connection goals and tracking your progress, as we did in the *Relationship Vitality Dashboard* in Chapter 3. Review these goals together weekly to celebrate successes, identify areas for improvement, and adjust your strategies accordingly. As you embrace strategy scaling, remember the purpose is successful, lasting and deeply fulfilling couple connection.

Your Action Steps:

Take time with your partner to ponder the *Reflection* Questions above, appreciating your love habits that are working well, and thinking what else will help you amplify or scale your success. Use your metrics to celebrate how far you have come and to extend your SMARTAR goals.

COUPLE STORIES ILLUSTRATING LEVERAGE

Maximized Medical Couple Moments

Zach and Ava examined and enlarged their established patterns with professional precision:

- Their morning chai ritual expanded to include a shared gratitude practice
- Their hospital corridor passes now involved subtle hand signals for emotional state
- Their evening routine incorporated elements from both their cultural traditions

"We're not changing what works," Ava noted. "We're amplifying it. Like increasing the signal strength of something already broadcasting clearly."

The Tea Ceremony Engineers

In their Osaka apartment, Yuki watched Hamish adjust their morning tea ritual with the precision he brought to his aerospace engineering. What had begun as a simple connection point had evolved into something both ancient and new.

"Look," Hamish explained, showing her his notebook. "When we add the moment of silence before whisking the matcha, our whole morning flows better. And if we position our cushions at this exact angle..." He demonstrated how the slight change created both intimacy and ease.

Yuki smiled, recalling her nana's delight at how this Scottish engineer had taken her traditional lessons and optimized them without losing their soul. "You've turned our tea ceremony into a launch sequence," she teased gently. "But isn't it?" Hamish replied, measuring the perfect water temperature. "Each successful connection lays the launchpad for the next flight."

"In the end," as Hamish told Yuki over their perfectly timed tea ceremony, "we're not just optimizing moments. We're optimizing our ability to be present for each other. And that's the greatest system upgrade of all, especially with our baby on the way."

CLOSING REFLECTION AND SUCCESS STORY

The Final Refinement

As the sun set over Santiago, Ava and Zach reviewed their optimized connection system. "It's not about adding more," Ava noted, "it's about making what we have count more."

Zach nodded, thinking of his surgical procedures. "Like how a single precise incision works better than multiple approximate ones." They'd learned that leveraging couple connection by relationship optimization wasn't about perfection but presence. Each refined moment, each amplified connection point or enhanced ritual added to their growing legacy of love.

Remember: Optimizing connection points isn't about mechanical efficiency but deepening intimacy. Like master craftspeople refining their art, each small improvement or thoughtful enhancement builds something greater than the sum of its parts.

Key Takeaway 9: Optimizing successful approaches maximizes relationship growth.

In Chapter Ten, *DEEPEN – Architecture Strengthening,* we will help you systematically bolster your practices and routines to ensure lasting change.

10

DEEPEN - ARCHITECTURE STRENGTHENING

We are what we repeatedly do. Excellence, then, is not an act, but a habit

— ARISTOTLE

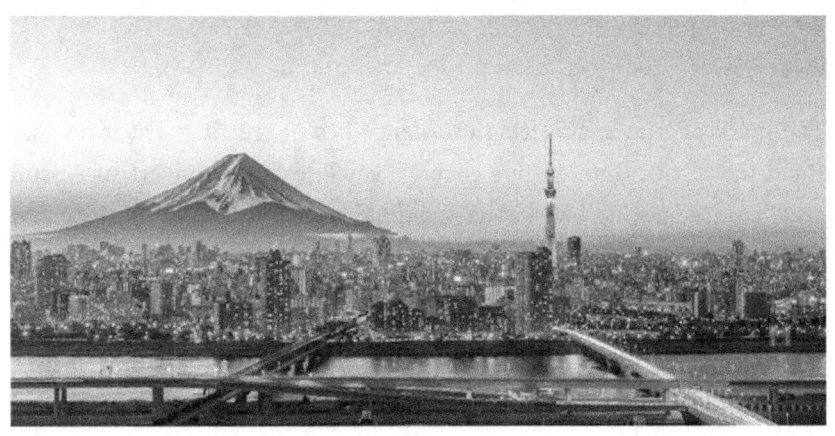

Real Life Scenario: The Earthquake Engineers

The Tokyo dawn painted Mount Fuji pink as Keiko felt the first tremor. Beside her, Chen stirred semi-asleep, his structural engineer's instincts reacting even before consciousness. Years of living on the Pacific Ring of Fire had taught them - some foundations strengthen under pressure.

"Remember the 2011 tsunami?" Keiko whispered as they fully awoke. *"How we learnt that rigid buildings shatter, but flexible ones survive?"* Chen nodded, pulling her closer, both of them thinking of the coastal towns they'd helped rebuild since then.

"Our love is like that," he said softly. *"Each challenge makes us more flexible, more resilient. Not because we're unshakeable, but because we've learned to sway together."*

Resilient High-Achieving Couples Deepening Their Connection Often Ask:

- How do we celebrate, continue and build on our successes?
- How will we make this growth normal and sustainable?

Overview

The mark of true engineering excellence lies in creating structures that stand the test of time. In this chapter, you'll learn to convert successful practices into lasting love habits, building a relationship architecture that strengthens itself through daily operation.

Architecture strengthening isn't just maintaining what works - it's about creating self-reinforcing systems that naturally deepen connection over time. By integrating successful practices into your daily routine, you will build a relationship infrastructure that grows stronger through regular use, just like any well-engineered system.

Your strengthening process will:

- Turn successful practices into automatic behaviors
- Create self-sustaining connection cycles
- Build resilient relationship infrastructure
- Develop maintenance routines that ensure lasting stability

PRACTICE INTEGRATION

Imagine your relationship as a complex architectural structure, requiring thoughtful design and ongoing enhancement to remain resilient. Like skyscrapers withstand the forces of nature through meticulous engineering, your relationship thrives by integrating practices that reinforce its foundations. For many high-achieving couples, the demands of careers, family and personal growth can overshadow intentional relationship-building. However, like in architecture, the strength of your partnership lies in the details. Here - we build practice integration, weaving consistent, meaningful connection routines into your relationship for long-term resilience.

Integrating connection practices matters as much as embedding other healthy habits into your daily life. These activities seem small but yield great fruit – that feeds your bond. According to research by Campbell and Ponzetti (2007), rituals are powerful predictors of relationship commitment, keeping partners connected amidst the challenges of life.

Reviewing your *Connection Baseline* and how your *6-Minute Connects* are working is a great way to start practice integration. Along with how the timing of your *Best Connection Points* is serving you? *What is the quality of your Midday Check-ins and overall KCIs like right now?* Then scale how strong your *Trust, Intimacy and Communication* is, using the *TICS* and combine all these qualitative metrics into a summary score from 1-10, to rate your *Relationship Vitality*.

If you didn't enter those in your **Relationship Vitality Dashboard** in Chapter 3, go ahead and take the time to do that now. You'll be glad you did, as this will give you a one-stop-shop view of all the working parts of your couple connection. Keep recording metrics in your Dashboard, and use the blank templates in *Appendix A: Connection Assessment Tools*, to make more copies.

As you reflect on how well these connection practices are working so far, remember it is early days. Recall in *Kolb's Experiential Learning Cycle* (Chapter 5), that reflection and feedback from each other can help you refine your approach and enhance closeness. This iterative process mirrors agile development, where continuous refinement leads to optimal outcomes.

ROUTINE ESTABLISHMENT

For couples navigating career and family responsibilities, establishing relationship routines can act as a stabilizing force, providing a predictable structure for secure connection. If your relationship is a finely tuned machine, each part working in harmony to achieve a greater purpose, then routines serve as the gears that keep your partnership running smoothly. These are not mere schedules; they are intentional practices that prioritize your relationship.

Routine establishment involves conscious effort to align schedules and priorities. This proactive approach minimizes stress and reinforces your commitment to nurturing the relationship. When well aligned, you can integrate shared activities into your day more easily. Normalizing routines in your relationship creates a shared narrative that reflects your values and aspirations.

Moreover, routines should incorporate elements that promote physical, mental, and emotional well-being as you measured in our 'Whole of System Overview,' at the start. Engaging in joint wellness activities, like exercising together or practicing mindfulness, can amplify the benefits of routine establishment. These activities enhance your individual well-being and create shared experiences that strengthen your bond, benefiting your family, workplace and community.

Reflection Questions:

> # How well are your morning, midday and evening connection practices working at this stage?
> # What improvements have you noticed and enjoyed – that can be celebrated?
> # What would lift the quality of each connection time up one percentage point?

Remember, love is a verb, and the key is kind actions, done 'little and often,' to build enjoyable and unbreakable love. It is the quality, more than the duration of your connection times that will strengthen trust, deepen your emotional intimacy and improve communication.

SYSTEM MAINTENANCE

In high-performing relationships, maintaining systems that support your connection is like ensuring the infrastructure of a thriving city remains robust and efficient. System maintenance can be thought of as the ongoing care and attention required to keep the mechanisms of your relationship operating smoothly. For many couples, this entails regular check-ins and fine-tuning, like software updates that keep a program running efficiently. It's about being proactive, rather than reactive, ensuring small issues are addressed before they escalate into large ones.

A crucial part of system maintenance is regularly checking the health of your relationship like we did with your ***Key Connection Indicators (KCIs)***, and ***Trust, Intimacy and Communication Scale (TICS)***. Review these and if you haven't entered any scores in yet, have a chat and try it.

Your Action Steps:

Scale Your Trust, Intimacy and Communication Levels in Light of Your Metrics Above

Review your Metrics recorded earlier, then Rate with your partner the resulting quality of these three connection ingredients on our: *Trust, Intimacy and Communication Scale (TICS)*. Note: it is normal for partners to give different ratings on these vital signs – for shared discussion.

Trust Scale: 0 _____ 10 (10 = Best)
Intimacy Scale: 0 _____ 10
Communication Scale: 0 _____ 10

RELATIONSHIP VITALITY SCALE: 0 _____ 10 (10 = Best)

Now Combine your Metrics, Connection KCIs and TIC Scale to Rate Your Resulting:

Regular **KCIs** conversations are as valuable as the lights on the dash of your car, giving you a basis for qualitatively measuring your *Relationship Vitality*.

Have you done that yet or are you concerned about what you might find?

No problem. The way to do it is to appreciate whatever score you get, then ask each other, *"What will lift us up one point? What will we do each day this week to help us improve?"*

Encouragement from your family and friends will also help, so hopefully you have recruited them as your raving fans by now.

Another aspect of effective system maintenance is growing emotional intelligence, like oiling your gears. This just means increasing your ability to understand and respond to your emotions and those of your partner. Emotional intelligence helps communication, empathy, and conflict resolution, essential for maintaining a strong connection. I recommend activities that grow these muscles - like useful books, podcasts, workshops and sharing one emotion daily at home. You could use the *How We Feel* App, to briefly keep track of your feelings and notice patterns.

$E=MH^2$ The Endurance and Enjoyment of any relationship (E), will be equivalent to the Mental Health (MH) of the two people in it

— DARYL PARSONS

System maintenance means nurturing intimacy and connection in spite of the busyness of life, so closeness retains a front seat. Systematizing love habits strengthens the lifeblood of your relationship, reinforcing your bond and reminding you of the love that brought you together.

Finally, remember that system maintenance is an ongoing process, not a one-time task. As a car requires regular servicing to function optimally, so your relationship needs consistent care and attention. Think about how maintaining and strengthening your couple connection systems can keep you strong, poised for growth and success together in the next phase of your journey.

CLOSING REFLECTION AND SUCCESS STORY

The Final Blueprint

As another tremor gentled through Tokyo, Keiko and Chen reviewed their relationship's architectural plans:

- Foundation: Deep cultural respect
- Support beams: Daily connection rituals
- Flexible joints: Adaptation strategies

- Safety features: Emotional safe spaces
- Maintenance schedule: Regular check-ins

"The strongest buildings," Chen observed, *"are the ones that are maintained the best and remember every storm they've survived."*

Key Takeaway 10: Systematic reinforcement ensures lasting change.

Remember: Love is a verb, and the key is kind actions, done 'little and often' to build enjoyable and unbreakable love.

Having recorded your couple metrics including your *KCIs*, *TICS* and *Relationship Vitality*, now we move on to Part 3 – FORTIFY. **In Chapter Eleven**, *Crisis-Proofing Your Connection*, we will show how to prepare your relationship to survive and hold steady in challenging times, equipping you with strategies to navigate life's inevitable obstacles with confidence and grace.

Your 28-Day Transformation Roadmap:

Week 1: Getting Started

- Day 1-3: Assessment ✅
- Day 4-7: Goal setting ✅
- Action focus: Morning rituals ✅

Week 2: Establishing Habits

- Day 8-14: Practice recording ✅
- Implementation focus: Daytime connection ✅
- Family rhythm integration ✅

Week 3: Optimizing Connection

- Day 15-21: System optimization ✅
- Strategic refinement: Evening habits ✅

- Family adaptation support

Week 4: Consolidation and Celebration

- Day 22-28: Success amplification
- Sustainable integration: Routine set
- Longterm connection enhancement

MAKE A DIFFERENCE WITH YOUR REVIEW - UNLOCK COUPLE CONNECTION FOR OTHERS

"A strong relationship isn't built in a day - it's built every day"

— UNKNOWN

Every relationship grows stronger with warm encouragement, and your words can make a real difference.

Would you help someone just like yourselves - an ambitious, analytically minded couple looking to reconnect but unsure where to start?

My mission is to make *Couple Connection Mastery* accessible to every couple seeking to strengthen their bond. But to reach more people, I need your help.

Most people choose books based on reviews. That means your review could be a key to helping more couples start on the path toward stronger trust, deeper intimacy and better communication. It takes one minute, but its impact could be life-changing.

Your review could help...

- ...one more couple turn distance into closeness.
- ...one more partnership engineer unbreakable love.
- ...one more family create a healthier happier home.
- ...one more dream of a thriving relationship come true.

To make a difference, simply scan the E-Book or Paper Back QR code below and leave a review

If you believe in the power of *Couple Connection*, you're my kind of person. Thank you from the bottom of my heart!

Daryl Parsons

PART III

FORTIFY

11

CRISIS-PROOFING YOUR CONNECTION

Don't wait until you're in a crisis to come up with a crisis plan

— PHIL MCGRAW

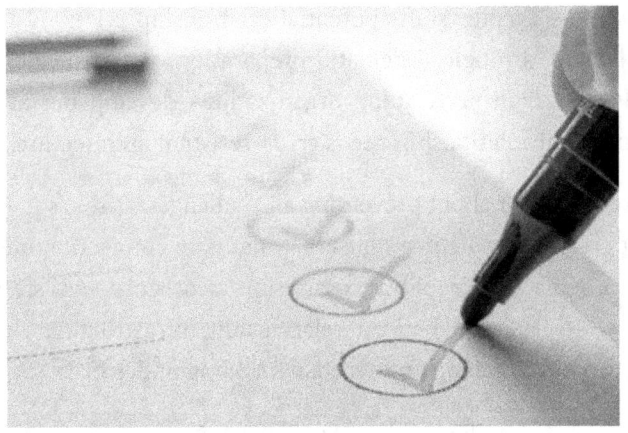

Real Life Scenario: Warning Systems in the Philippines

In Manila, Maria and James woke with phones buzzing for typhoon alerts. As meteorologists, they understood nature's warning systems. As partners, they'd developed their own.

"Remember our first super typhoon together?" Maria asked, checking their emergency supplies. *"How we thought being prepared meant just having enough food and water?"* James nodded, already sending updates to their extended family WhatsApp group. *"Now we know crisis-proofing is about more than physical supplies. It's about emotional preparation too."*

High-Performance Couples Planning for Contingencies in their Relationship Ask:

- What backup plans should we have for extremely tough times?
- What will help us to repair our bond when we feel disconnected?
- How do we maintain our connection during major life changes?

Overview

Every well-engineered system includes robust fail safes and emergency protocols. This chapter shifts potential relationship crises into manageable challenges through systematic preparation and strategic response design. Just as high-performing organizations develop business continuity plans, your relationship needs crisis-resistant architecture.

Crisis-proofing isn't about preventing all challenges, as that's not realistic. It's about creating resilient systems that maintain connection under pressure. By engineering rapid reconnection protocols and stress-tested bonding strategies, you build a relationship infrastructure that grows stronger through adversity, rather than buckling under it.

Through strategic crisis-proofing, you'll develop:

- Emergency response systems to hold together under pressure

- Quick-recovery steps for immediate reconnection
- Stress-resistant communication methods
- Systematic approaches to relationship resilience

This advanced engineering ensures your connection stays strong, even when facing unexpected challenges or high-stress periods.

WHY CRISIS-PROOFING YOUR CONNECTION MATTERS

Many high-achievers, handling the interplay of career success and personal fulfilment, are adept at problem-solving, managing teams, and innovating solutions at work. Yet, when faced with a crisis in their relationship - like unexpected job loss or family health emergency - they feel ill-equipped to apply the same strategic thinking to the challenges of their union.

In times of crisis, the stability of any relationship is tested, exposing vulnerabilities that may have been masked by the routine of daily life. In these moments having emergency response procedures is as vital as having steps to troubleshoot a critical system failure at work. By planning for relational disruptions, you can learn to navigate challenges with resilience and grace, ensuring your connection remains robust even in adversity.

Emergency Response Protocols

Emergency response protocols in a relationship are akin to a well-prepared contingency plan, designed to address the emotional and practical challenges that arise during crises. These protocols provide clarity and direction when emotions run high and cloud decision-making. In the heat of a crisis, misunderstandings can escalate tensions, making it essential to have pre-agreed methods of communication that bring clarity and empathy.

I recommend *Midday Check-ins* during testing times, so you each express your feelings and concerns in a safe, supportive space. We have found these so helpful as a couple. These check-ins can include active listening, validation of emotions, and collaborative problem-solving.

In addition to communication strategies, emergency response protocols must address the logistical challenges of a crisis. This may mean delegating tasks, adjusting priorities, and temporarily reallocating household chores to ease pressure on one or both partners.

It is also wise to have a support network in place, comprising trusted friends, family or professionals who can help when needed. By proactively identifying available resources, you ensure aid is readily accessible when required. See more on this in Chapter 14 and 15.

DESIGNING YOUR EMERGENCY RESPONSE PROTOCOLS

Spend time with your partner discussing potential crises that could impact your relationship.

Develop a set of emergency response protocols including communication strategies, logistical adjustments, and support systems. Write a plan to serve as a guide during challenging times and commit to refining your protocols regularly.

Here in Christchurch, New Zealand, we practice earthquake drills in anticipation of the Alpine Fault rupturing with a mega-quake over 8.0 on the Richter scale. This helps us plan in advance to cope with couple crises, as we have an existing model. Our physical preparation includes our civil defence kit, barbeque, non-perishable food and water supplies to last three days.

What natural disaster drills do you already have to guide your relational crisis preparedness?

Doing the physical practice and building your confidence with these emergency drills can equip you to manage future emotional challenges with strength and unity.

RAPID RECONNECTION TECHNIQUES

In the bustle of daily life, moments of disconnection occur unexpectedly, leaving you feeling distant from your partner. Such moments are natural, yet can cause anxiety if not addressed. This is why rapid reconnection matters, to bridge the emotional gap quickly and effectively.

Imagine a scenario where you've both had long days, filled with work and family demands. You are at the dinner table, but instead of engaging, you're absorbed in your thoughts or devices. This is a good opportunity to use a one-minute reconnection technique called the 'E-Check.'

Try an *E-Check* here. Pause, put down distractions, and share *three E's*, as follows.

The first E is your *Energy* right now, out of 100%, e.g. 45%. The second E is one *Emotion* that you feel right now, e.g tired. The third E is the resultant *Expectation* you have. Or *what do you need? For example, "With 45% energy and feeling tired, I need..?"* Then swap. We've done this as a family for years and it works. E-Checks let you know what space you are in and what could help.

Another powerful practice is 'The Gratitude Exchange.' It's easy to see what's lacking when stress levels are high. Instead, take turns giving thanks for something your partner did today. Even if it is just the small things, like making coffee or picking up the kids, this can shift the focus from silence or criticism to appreciation. Simple acts of gratitude can refresh the emotional climate, reinforce the positive and remind you of your mutually supportive bond.

Physical touch is another immediate way to reconnect, like you have practiced with the **6MC**. A gentle touch, like holding hands or a brief hug, can release oxytocin, the hormone associated with bonding and trust. Try the 'Two-Minute Touch' technique. Set aside 120 seconds to hold each other silently. This act of physical closeness warms hearts and builds a sense of safety.

For those who are geographically distant and so inclined, digital tools can serve reconnection. The *'Photo Share'* is sending a picture that captures a real moment in your day, whether it's a beautiful sunset or a funny meme. This visual exchange adds a layer of intimacy, allowing you to share experiences when apart. It provides a talking point for later conversations too.

At times, silence can be golden. The *'Shared Silence'* practice means sitting together quietly in a calm part of your home or in nature. This shared silence allows for reflection and a deeper sense of presence, creating space where words aren't needed to feel reconnected.

Incorporating these rapid reconnection methods into your daily routine ensures that moments of disconnection do not last. They take little time yet offer rich returns in emotional closeness, reminding you that connection is a choice - that can be reaffirmed with intention and care.

STRESS-TESTED BONDING STRATEGIES

In the high-octane world where success is measured by precise execution and thriving under pressure, the same applies to couple relationships. Picture your connection as a dynamic entity that, when stress-tested, shows its true strength and adaptability. This isn't about waiting for crises to strike but proactively building a bond tough enough to resist life's inevitable trials. Stress-tested bonding strategies fortify your connection on purpose, ensuring it stays steadfast when external pressures mount.

At the heart of these strategies is the understanding that shared challenges are opportunities for growth and deeper connection. Along with the above techniques, engaging in activities that require collaboration and problem-solving cultivates a sense of unity and interdependence.

A paradoxical aspect of stress-tested bonding involves seeing vulnerability as a strength rather than a weakness. Vulnerability is often viewed as a liability, yet in relationships, it is a powerful tool for connection. Sharing your fears, anxieties, and aspirations with your partner invites empathy and understanding, forging an emotional intimacy that can handle the fire of testing.

Physical wellness is another pillar of stress-tested bonding. Prioritize activities that promote physical health, like regular exercise, balanced nutrition, and adequate rest. Shared activities – like hiking, cycling, or a fitness class - strengthen your bond through joint experiences. Bodily health boosts individual well-being and the relational dynamic, as partners who feel physically capable are better equipped to manage stress and engage meaningfully with each other.

Lastly, laughter is a potent antidote to stress, so be humorous together and find brief moments to share joy and levity. Whether it's doing a silly dance, watching a comedy, playing a game, or sharing funny stories, laughter diffuses tension, releases endorphins and creates a sense of camaraderie. These light moments remind you that your relationship is a source of joy and fulfilment, despite the challenges. Use these strategies often to thicken your bond.

SUCCESS STORY: THE PANDEMIC PIVOT

Maria and James' progress: *"Covid taught us to build systems that bend but don't break. Now we have: Weekly outdoor family councils; monthly financial check-ins; quarterly care planning for our parents; and our annual cultural celebration calendar."*

Their Solution - The 'Whole Life Integration System' Encompassing:

Morning Unity Practice

- 5-minute prayer/meditation together
- Gratitude sharing
- Cultural wisdom moment
- Nature appreciation

146 | CRISIS-PROOFING YOUR CONNECTION

Daily Connection Points

- WhatsApp family group check-ins
- Shared responsibility tracking
- Crisis management protocols
- Joy moment documentation

Closing Reflection - The Storm Chasers

Maria and James had developed what they called their *'Typhoon Protocols,'* but these went far beyond standard emergency procedures:

"Watch this," Maria explained to their new colleague during a late-night monitoring shift. She typed a simple "🌀" into their private chat. Within moments, James responded with "🏠💜" which was their emoji shorthand for, *"I'm heading home, holding you in my heart."*

"During Typhoon Haiyan," she shared, *"we learned that crisis communication needs to be both efficient and emotional. One symbol can carry an entire conversation's worth of love."*

Around the world, couples are discovering that true crisis-proofing means:

- Building systems before they're needed
- Regular testing and refinement
- Flexible response protocols
- Deep trust in foundations

Whether facing natural disasters, family emergencies, illness, career challenges, or personal struggles, crisis-proofed relationships share common elements:

- Clear communication systems
- Practiced response protocols
- Emotional safety measures

- Basic recovery routines
- Shared wisdom stories

As the sun set over Manila Bay, Maria sent her simple, "🌀" signal. James' reply "🏠❤️" came back instantly. Another storm was coming, but their connection was ready.

Key Takeaway 11: Prepared couples maintain connection through any challenge.

Remember: *"The secret,"* as Maria and James would say during their Manila typhoon briefings, *"isn't avoiding crises - it's building a connection so strong it can weather any storm."*

In Chapter Twelve, *Long-Distance Engineering*, we refine digital and other remote bonding practices to ensure connection strategies make distance relating more meaningful.

12

LONG-DISTANCE ENGINEERING

Let there be spaces in your togetherness

— KAHLIL GIBRAN

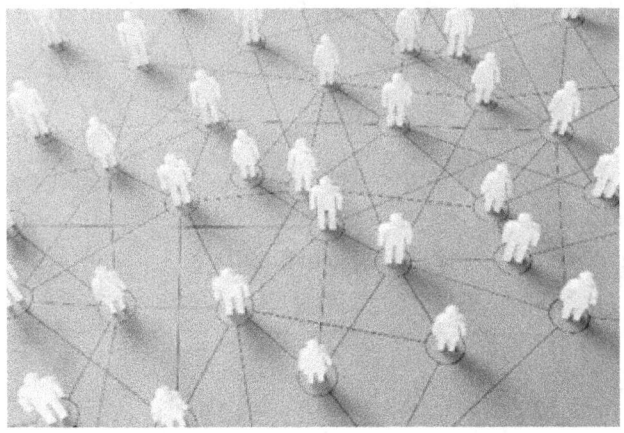

Real Life Scenario: The Pacific Bridge Between Hawaii and Auckland

Working far away from his beloved was a familiar experience now for marine biologist Kalani, stationed two months at a time in Hawaii, then two months back in New Zealand with his veterinary scientist partner, Moana. Consequently, he cherished online connection like this.

"Some think the ocean is mostly empty but in truth - it is full of vast, connected ecosystems," Moana's dad had told her over the years. Now, standing at Auckland's North Shore while video calling Kalani in Oahu, Moana understood deeper truths about distance and connection.

"Tell me about your little blue penguins," Kalani encouraged her, his phone propped on a lab bench at the marine research station. Their daily ritual unfolded with sharing their hemisphere's stories across the international date line.

"They're starting to pair up for breeding season," Moana replied, watching waves pattern the sand. *"Like us - finding ways to bond across seemingly impossible distances."*

High-Performance Couples Doing Distance-Relating Have Questions Like:

- How do we handle connection points during travel or separation?
- How do we prevent future disconnection when living in two countries?
- What systems can we use to ensure our bond keeps growing stronger?

Overview

Physical distance doesn't have to mean emotional distance when applying love engineering. This chapter shows how virtual connection systems can maintain intimacy across any gap. For couples facing travel demands or remote work situations, such strategies are essential.

Long-distance connection isn't about compensating for absence, but engineering channels for intimacy that can at times serve better than in-person approaches. By designing systematic digital connection points and virtual bonding protocols, you create a relationship architecture that thrives regardless of physical proximity.

Your long-distance engineering will:

- Turn virtual interactions into powerful connection points
- Hone digital intimacy systems to transcend physical distance
- Plan time zone-optimized communication protocols
- Strengthen location-independent bonding practices

THE VALUE OF LONG-DISTANCE ENGINEERED LOVE

Imagine standing on opposite sides of a vast canyon, your voices echoing across the chasm, yet being unable to close the distance by one step. This metaphor depicts the reality faced by many couples traversing long-distance relationships, where career opportunities and personal commitments require physical separation. This can make it difficult to maintain a thriving relationship. However, just as skilled engineers construct bridges to span great divides, you can use virtual connection to sustain and enrich your relationship, despite the miles between you.

VIRTUAL CONNECTION DESIGN

Using technology to nurture emotional intimacy and effectively span the gap between partners, is an art. Thoughtfully leveraging digital tools can help replicate the warmth of face-to-face interactions. The key is a range of communication methods that cater to your needs, ensuring the digital bridge you build is as strong as the love it supports. I suggest use of various apps and platforms that support your unique relationship, via communication and shared experiences.

Many couples schedule brief video calls to engage in meaningful conversation and share nonverbal cues that cannot be felt via text communication. This visual immediacy can foster shared presence and space to discuss daily events and challenges. Video calls can also be used creatively for virtual date nights, where you can cook the same meal, watch a movie simultaneously, or even take a virtual walk through a city using online maps. Such shared activities help maintain a sense of togetherness and strengthen your emotional bond.

Beyond video calls, explore creatively using voice messages and texts to maintain consistent lines of communication during the day. These brief interactions show support to your partner. Try apps like *Paired*, which offer daily questions and games to spark meaningful conversations, or *Love Nudge*, which lets you send affectionate messages and reminders. These tools provide ways to emotionally connect, ensuring your partner feels valued and appreciated from afar.

To thicken your virtual connection, consider creating shared digital spaces to document and celebrate your relationship. A shared photo album or digital journal helps you capture moments and memories, making a visual narrative of your partnership. Apps like *MyLove*, which track relationship milestones, provide a sense of continuity and progression together.

Virtual connection is an ongoing process requiring intentionality, creativity, and adaptability. By embracing the available tools and integrating them thoughtfully into your relationship, you can transcend space and time, ensuring your love remains as vibrant and fulfilling as if you were side by side. Doing this purposefully will increase the depth of your commitment to one another.

REMOTE INTIMACY BUILDING

For couples separated by geography, building remote closeness is vital. This involves cultivating a sense of bonding and understanding despite the distance. The key to remote intimacy lies in the ability to share experiences, thoughts, and emotions as if there were no miles in between. Technology then serves your relationship as a bridge and a backdrop, providing the tools needed to maintain this connection while you keep interactions genuine and heartfelt.

One effective practice in nurturing remote intimacy is shared virtual experiences, like reading the same book and discussing it day by day to provide a shared narrative and a sense of unity. Choose experiences that resonate with you both, so activities are enjoyable and meaningful.

Another valued part of remote intimacy building is regular sharing of insights and reflections. More than updating your partner on your day, this means by disclosing your thoughts, feelings, and aspirations. Some write a weekly letter or email to each other, expressing their learnings, hopes, or how they perceive the relationship evolving. These written exchanges hold emotional depth, capturing the essence of your connection in words. They allow for humorous musings and provide a tangible record of your journey, preserving the nuances of your relationship.

Lastly, cultivating truth and trust is the glue of remote intimacy building. This requires clear communication about your daily activities, plans and challenges. Transparency mitigates the potential for misunderstandings and builds a solid sense of security. It is in these conversations that the seeds of trust are grown, allowing intimacy to flourish in the fertile ground of honesty.

DIGITAL BONDING PROTOCOLS

In the age of virtual interconnectedness, forging robust digital bonding protocols is crucial for couples separated by distance. This requires structured yet flexible strategies that leverage technology to maintain your relationship's emotional core. At the heart of digital bonding is the intentional and consistent use of technology that helps you both feel prioritized and valued.

Beyond planned interactions, spontaneity can breathe life into digital communication. Sending a surprise message or meme that reminds you of your partner can build a sense of immediacy and presence. These small gestures can reinforce your affection, showing your partner that they are central in your thoughts. Additionally, consider using apps designed to facilitate connection.

These tools, like those offering shared timelines or playlists, involve elements of common experience, helping you engage in activities simultaneously, bridging the physical divide with mutual enjoyment. Apps like *Gottman Card Decks* can also be instrumental, offering prompts that spark deeper conversations, enhancing your emotional understanding of each other.

Digital bonding protocols must allow for resolving conflicts. Disagreements are inevitable, and distance can exacerbate misunderstandings, so establishing a method for conflict resolution is essential. This may involve agreeing to pause a heated discussion until you're both calmer, or setting a rule to address issues as they arise, stopping resentment from brewing. Using video calls for this can enhance empathy by seeing facial expressions and body language.

Digital bonding protocols offer ways to maintain vibrant connection despite physical separation. As you explore these strategies, consider how they fit in the broader space of your relationship, ensuring that your bond remains as dynamic and rewarding as your professional achievements.

Action Steps

1. Today
    - Map your time zones
    - Identify prime connection windows
    - Set up primary communication tools
    - Create emergency protocols
2. This Week
    - Establish daily check-in rituals
    - Test all backup systems
    - Plan next virtual date
    - Contact support crew
3. This Month
    - Review and adjust timing
    - Upgrade connection tools
    - Strengthen support systems
    - Celebrate small wins

Reflection Questions:

What would help improve the quality and enjoyment of your remote intimacy?

How are you planning to constructively handle conflicts and disagreements?

Who else is in your support crew or top three trusted people while you are apart?

Measuring Long-Distance Success

Along with the *E-Checks* mentioned earlier, you can use adapted versions of your **6MC** and **Midday Check-in**, tracking metrics like your **KCIs** and **TICS** fortnightly in your **Dashboard** to keep an eye on your **Relationship Vitality** while working and living in different locations.

CLOSING REFLECTION

As the sun sets over Auckland, Moana and Kalani review their weekly metrics via video call while drinking the same tea on opposite sides of the Pacific Ocean. *"Our sciences have taught us precision in measuring connection,"* Kalani reflects, *"but love taught us how to deeply connect in spite of distance. Using the separateness well actually improves our togetherness in person."*

Key Takeaway 12: Distance becomes irrelevant with engineered connection strategies.

Remember: Like sophisticated satellite systems, couples separated by oceans or orbits mix precise engineering with profound humanity to strengthen long-distance relationships.

In Chapter Thirteen, *Career-Connection Integration* - we'll see how couples blend professional success with relationship depth, building careers that support their connection. We will explore how the lessons of long-distance love can strengthen partnerships when working side by side.

13

CAREER-CONNECTION INTEGRATION

When love and skill work together, expect a masterpiece

— JOHN RUSKIN

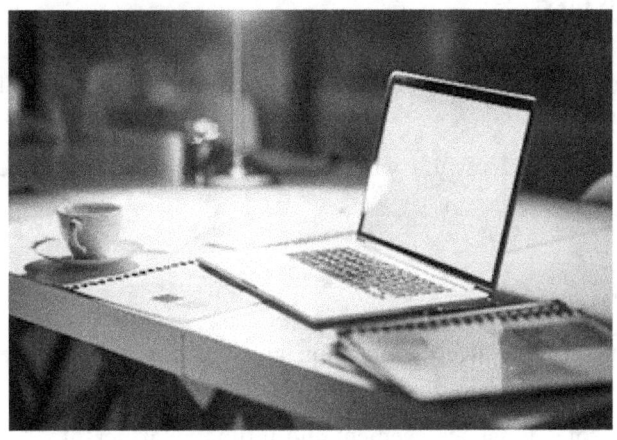

Real Life Scenario: Hospital Harmony in Chile

"Time of death, 3:47 AM," Dr. Zach recorded quietly, while across the Santiago hospital campus in the neo-natal ward, his wife Dr. Ava Rodriguez guided a newborn baby into the world. They'd learned to finely weave their medical careers and marriage into a beautiful tapestry of care.

"Remember our residency years?" Ava would ask during their precious cafeteria overlaps. "When we thought we had to choose between being good doctors and good partners?"

Now they'd engineered their connection around two demanding medical careers:

- Synchronized surgery schedules where possible
- Sacred chai moments between shifts or rounds
- Code words for emotional support during tough cases
- Shared celebration rituals for lives saved

High-Performance Professional Couples Integrating Careers Ask Questions Like:

- How will we maintain professional focus while improving our relationship?
- How do we successfully work, parent our children and connect as a couple?

Overview

Career success and deep connection aren't opposing forces when you engineer suitable integration systems. This chapter builds synergy between professional achievement and intimate partnership, turning the tension into opportunities for mutual growth.

Integration engineering isn't about compromise – it's about designing systems where career and connection amplify each other. With clear boundaries and strategic bonding, your professional success and relationship depth become mutually reinforcing rather than competing priorities.

Your integrated system will help you:

- Set professional boundaries that protect relationship vitality
- Make work-home synergy points that benefit both areas
- Form career strategies that enhance rather than diminish connection
- Develop protocols for maintaining intimacy during peak career demands

Career-Connection Integration - Costs and Benefits

In life's vibrant ecosystem, career goals and relationships can coexist in a delicate equilibrium, thanks to the quintessential art of integration. For high-performing couples, the trick is not in choosing between career and connection, but how to weave both into a harmonious tapestry. This chapter explains the strategies necessary for integrating career and connection.

PROFESSIONAL BOUNDARY SETTING

In this era where technology blurs the line between work and home, setting clear professional boundaries is essential for maintaining healthy relationships. As a therapist, I often see how the erosion of traditional work hours in favor of constant connectivity leads to stress and burnout, reduced emotional well-being and relationship distance. Understanding and setting boundaries is crucial to preserving not only job satisfaction but also personal connection.

Effectiveness requires negotiating specific work hours and clear expectations with workmates or managers about availability, then utilizing tools like away messages or status updates. Strong communication serves as the backbone of effective boundary setting, hence stating your needs and limitations candidly aids mutual agreement and prevents potential conflicts. Saying *"yes"* only when you genuinely mean it builds trust by aligning actions with words.

Responding to boundary crossings in real-time is a key part of boundary setting. When work demands threaten to overshadow personal plans or affect your health, addressing these promptly demonstrates self-respect and assertiveness. This can mean politely declining tasks outside your job description, rescheduling meetings that would infringe on your home time, or taking Sick Leave to have a few Mental Health days for recovery and reconnection.

Professional boundary setting is not just about creating separation between work and home but fostering a sustainable integration that respects both. By establishing clear boundaries, you empower yourselves to master the complexities of your work while growing couple connection.

WORK-HOME SYNERGY CREATION

In high-performance living, the idea of synergy between work and home has gained prominence. It transcends the traditional notion of balance since that suggested a zero-sum game where gains in one area meant losses in another. Synergy, however, emphasizes the complementary nature of work and home, highlighting the potential for each to enhance the other. For couples immersed in demanding careers, creating synergy is not just beneficial – it empowers you to cultivate lives where career ambitions and personal relationships coexist harmoniously.

The role of open communication cannot be overstated in creating synergy. Regular talks about each other's needs, priorities, and challenges enable alignment and understanding. Speaking candidly allows you to navigate conflicts, celebrate achievements, and recalibrate efforts.

You can make tech serve your work-home synergy, leveraging digital tools to streamline tasks, coordinate schedules, and share responsibilities to enhance efficiency and reduce stress.

Finally, nurturing work-home synergy requires a commitment to self-care. Prioritizing your physical, mental, and emotional health is essential for maintaining the energy and focus needed to thrive in all dimensions of well-being. This includes regular exercise, mindfulness practices, and carving out time for relaxation. By investing in your well-being, you enhance your own resilience while contributing to the strength and vitality of your relationship.

WINNING WITH ACHIEVEMENT AND INTIMACY

For high-performing couples, the pursuit of career milestones runs parallel with the desire for a deeply connected partnership, like parallel railway tracks. *If you assume career achievement and intimacy are mutually compatible, then approach them intentionally.* I commonly see the drive for professional excellence eclipsing the nurturing of emotional intimacy in my couple therapy clients. The key to thriving in both lies not in choosing one over the other, but in harmonizing them to create a cohesive life experience.

To achieve this, couples must value the emotional richness intimacy brings to the rest of their lives. Intimacy, characterized by vulnerability, trust, and emotional support, offers a refuge from the stress of career pursuits. In this safe space individuals find the strength to recharge and face professional challenges with renewed vigor. Emotional nourishment from a strong, intimate partnership catalyzes creativity and resilience at work, enabling individuals to traverse complex professional landscapes with confidence. *Thus, investing in intimacy is not a diversion from career goals but a strategic enhancement of one's overall effectiveness and well-being.*

Ultimately, the balance between achievement and intimacy is not a static state but an ongoing process of negotiation and recalibration. It requires a conscious effort to prioritize and integrate career and connection, recognizing that each enriches the other in profound ways.

Action Steps

1. Today

   - Choose one connection point to improve
   - Track this on your *Relationship Dashboard*
   - Discuss and agree on plans with your partner
   - Record this connection data in your *Dashboard*

2. This Week

   - Review daily check-in metrics
   - Assess career-connection levels
   - Review initial data together
   - Adjust tracking as needed

3. This Month

   - Analyze trends in your data
   - Celebrate measurable wins
   - Refine tracking systems
   - Plan next integration level

Success Metrics: Include Career Integration in Your Relationship Dashboard

Track these Key Indicators:

1. Connection Quality

   - Daily touch points completed
   - Meaningful exchanges achieved

- Support moments offered
- Celebration rituals shared

2. Career Support

   - Professional celebrations shared
   - Work challenges processed
   - Growth goals aligned
   - Success strategies shared

3. Integration Effectiveness

   - Schedule coordination rate
   - Crisis response success
   - Innovation sharing benefits
   - Relationship satisfaction trend

SUCCESS STORIES: HOW TWO COUPLES TRACKED THEIR PROGRESS

The Hospital 6MC Check-In System

Zach & Ava developed their 'Vital Signs Chart' by adapting their *6MC* love habit to suit their work. *"Just like patient monitoring,"* Zach explained during their cafeteria break, *"we rate each connection point on a simple 1-5 scale: 1 = Missed connection; 2 = Brief acknowledgment; 3 = Quick emotional check-in; 4 = Meaningful exchange; and 5 = Deep connection moment."*

They tracked three touch points daily:

- Morning huddle (target score: 4+)
- Midday signal (target score: 2+)
- Evening debrief (target score: 4+)

"*Over a week,*" Ava added, showing their simple notes APP, "*we aim for an average of 3.5. That's how we got our 71% emotional support metric - we hit or exceeded our target 71% of the time.*"

Summarizing Two Couples' Success: The Hospital Heroes and Engineering Excellence

Zach & Ava achieved:

- Daily connection rate: 71%
- Career support satisfaction: 84%
- Work-home integration: 79% Through their simple vital signs tracking system

Keiko and Chen maintained:

- Project collaboration: 73%
- Relationship strength: 78%
- Crisis management: 85% Using their earthquake-proof relationship metrics

Key Takeaway 13: Career success and deep connection can coexist harmoniously when couples show the same wholehearted dedication in their relationship as they do at their work.

CLOSING REFLECTION

As Zach shared, "*Ava and I learnt how to integrate our careers satisfactorily with our couple and family priorities by intentionally working on it together. This works as long as we measure and review how we are going weekly and give each other grace for the variables that occur each day.*"

Remember: Achieving harmony between work and home is a dynamic process, requiring ongoing effort and intentionality. Couples can bring their professional excellence home and their relationship wisdom to work, to make something greater than either may achieve alone.

In Chapter Fourteen, *Family System Integration*, we help couples maintain their connection while nurturing complex families. We'll see how the measurement systems and professional wisdom we've developed can strengthen not just partnerships, but entire kinship groups.

14

FAMILY SYSTEM INTEGRATION

In family life and parenting, love is often spelt: T. I. M. E

— IAN GRANT

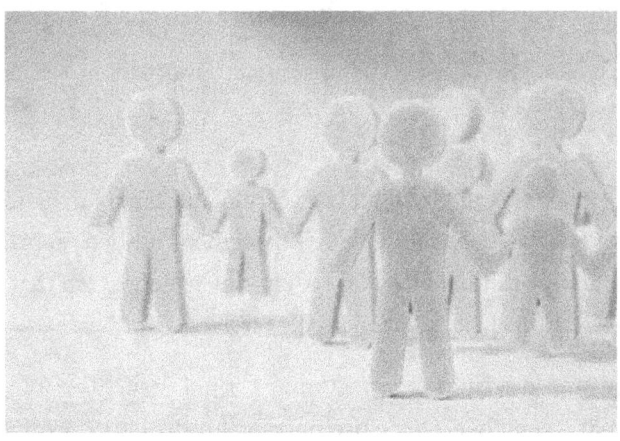

Real Life Scenario - The Birthday Reality Check

Remember Hamish and Yuki's *'kintsugi'* tea bowl repair earlier? Here's another real family event.

Thabo and Amara's Daughter's 13th Birthday in Johannesburg

Birthday Plans	Reality	Connection Score
Traditional breakfast	Slept late, rushed	1/5
School celebration	Forgot cupcakes	0/5
Family gathering	Teen mood swing	2/5
Special dinner	Restaurant closed	1/5
Evening ritual	Unexpected tears, real talk	5/5

"That last moment," Thabo shared, *"when everything had 'failed' - that's when we had our deepest connection. She finally told us how scared she was, growing up between two cultures."*

High-Performance Couples Feeling Family Pressures Often Ask:

- How can we reach agreement about how we parent and manage family expectations?
- How do we strengthen our relationship and wider family bonds whilst setting limits?

Overview

Complex systems require careful integration and family dynamics are no exception. Here we promote and strengthen unified approaches to extended family relationships and parenting challenges, so that potential stress points are utilized for deeper partnership.

Family integration isn't about enforcing rigid structures but creating systems that strengthen your core partnership while managing external relationships effectively. Making clear protocols and united front strategies can help your connection grow stronger amid family challenges.

Through systematic family integration, you'll:

- Better align parenting systems that strengthen your partnership
- Make efficient protocols for managing extended family dynamics
- Sharpen united front strategies that protect your connection
- Develop family decision-making habits that enhance intimacy

PARENTING PARTNERSHIP ALIGNMENT

The pulse of every thriving family is a heartbeat with individual and collective beats, a rhythm of roles and responsibilities that, when harmonized, creates a resilient and nurturing environment. For high-achieving couples, the challenge often lies in synchronizing the demands of their professional ambitions with the dynamics of their family lives.

Parenting Partnership Alignment

In the morphing world of parenting, aligning as partners is vital for handling the complexities of raising children. Amidst the myriad responsibilities of life, strong parenting teamwork not only fosters a nurturing environment for children but also strengthens the partner bond.

One of the most effective practices in achieving alignment involves turning towards each other in moments of need. This means recognizing and responding to bids for support (central to the Gottman Method) thereby maintaining emotional connection amidst the chaos of parenting. When disagreements arise, using constructive conflict resolution techniques like soft start-ups and repair attempts, can deescalate misunderstandings. These strategies not only preserve harmony but also model healthy communication for your children.

Shared parenting goals are another cornerstone of a successful partnership. Within regular family meetings, you can set SMARTAR goals, recording these on vision boards or action plans, to help everyone get on the same page. Regular check-ins further reinforce this, providing opportunities to celebrate successes, address challenges, and recalibrate goals as needed. We do these meetings every Sunday night and it helps us to be organized and care for each other.

Expressing appreciation and positive affirmation plays a significant role in building a positive parenting culture. By acknowledging each other's contributions and expressing gratitude for small acts of kindness, you create an atmosphere of mutual respect and support.

Engaging in family fun times further solidifies your partnership, creating a strong family identity. Whether it's joining in a community event, hiking in nature, playing games or simply enjoying meals together, these shared experiences build a sense of team and common purpose. They provide spaces for connection and joy, essential ingredients in a thriving family system.

Reflection Section:

Take a moment to reflect on your current parenting partnership.

In what areas are you strongly aligned and what requires further attention?

Discuss together any challenges or aspirations you have and explore how the principles in this chapter can be applied to enhance your partnership.

List your shared parenting goals, action steps and plan regular check-ins to notice progress.

EXTENDED FAMILY NAVIGATION

For couples juggling careers and personal commitments, extended family can be both a source of support and a potential stressor. The key lies in clear communication and setting healthy boundaries that honor the needs of both your immediate family and your close relatives.

According to research, clear communication can significantly reduce misunderstandings and prevent the conflicts escalating. This involves being assertive yet compassionate, expressing your thoughts and feelings without blaming or making assumptions about others' intentions.

Clear boundaries help maintain functional relationships with extended family, delineating roles and responsibilities, limiting conflicts that arise from unmet expectations or encroachment on personal space. Setting boundaries requires truthful talk about what you are comfortable with as a couple, like frequency of visits, decision-making, or sharing of personal information.

When managing unsolicited advice from well-meaning relatives, it's important to approach these interactions with empathy and patience. Such advice often stems from a place of love and concern, rather than criticism. By acknowledging the intent behind it, you can respond with gratitude and assert your own view respectfully. Their response is their responsibility.

Incorporating extended family into your life can also enrich your family's cultural and social experiences. Engaging in shared traditions like celebrating cultural holidays, family reunions, or feasts can create lasting memories of interconnectedness in your family network. Proactively involving extended family in your life grows a supportive community that can offer care, help, guidance, and companionship.

However, it's equally important to recognize when to prioritize your immediate family's needs over those of your extended family. This can mean making hard choices to protect your time, energy, and emotional well-being. By negotiating these, and often reaching a compromise, you can agree how to approach family dynamics. This will strengthen your partnership and set a positive example for your children, to balance familial obligations with personal well-being.

If things get stuck, seek professional guidance such as family counseling. This can help you keep sane while being reasonable with your extended family - as far as it depends on you.

UNITED FRONT ENGINEERING

As couples handle the demands of life, standing together as a cohesive unit is so important. The notion of a united front extends beyond mere agreement; it embodies a shared commitment to approach challenges with a unified perspective, reinforcing the strength of the partnership.

The process of engineering a united front begins with establishing shared values and goals that serve to guide decision-making, ensuring both partners are agreed in their parenting, finances, friendships, time use and other parts of a shared life. Honest communication is key for the exploration of differences and identification of common ground.

In practice, presenting a united front involves supporting each other's decisions and shows a willingness to prioritize the partnership over individual preferences, recognizing that the strength of the relationship is paramount. It requires patience and humility, acknowledging that neither partner has all the answers.

This means accepting that disagreements are natural. These are to be expected in any relationship and the true measure of your partnership lies in how you work through these with empathy and respect. By approaching conflicts as opportunities to grow, you can build safety and help each other feel valued and heard, reinforcing your couple bond.

Action Steps:

1. Today

    - Note one real family moment (good or bad)
    - Share one honest feeling about it
    - Make one small connection attempt
    - Accept whatever happens

2. This Week

- Track actual vs. planned family times
- Document both failures and successes
- Notice unexpected connection moments
- Celebrate small wins and recoveries

3. This Month

- Review your family's natural rhythms
- Adjust expectations to reality
- Build on what actually works
- Let go of perfectionist goals

Success Metrics - Track What Actually Matters:

Connection Type	Target	Acceptable Reality
Morning Ritual	Daily	3-4 times/week
Meals Together	Daily	When possible
Quality Talk	Daily	5 minutes still counts
Crisis Recovery	Perfect	Messy but honest

MEASURING FAMILY CONNECTION AND REPAIR PROCESSES IN FOUR OF OUR GLOBAL FAMILIES

The Intergenerational Bridge

In their Osaka home, Yuki and Hamish had blended Scottish and Japanese family traditions into what their children called 'The Family Festival Calendar.' As Yuki explained, *"Each month has its own connection theme,"* pointing to their beautifully illustrated wall chart. *"July combines Tanabata with Highland games - the kids learn both cultures through celebration."*

THEIR TRACKING SYSTEM WAS AN ELEGANTLY SIMPLE POSTER ON THE PANTRY:

- Cultural events shared: ★
- Family stories told: 💬
- Traditions blended: 🌀
- Memories documented: 📷

Real Family Rhythms with Thabo and Amara

One day of their actual weekly tracker of their *6-Minute Connects* showed:

Monday - Honest Connection Quality:

Morning rush: 2/5 (Kids cranky, missed connection)

Afternoon check-in: 0/5 (Work crisis, forgot)

Evening gathering: 4/5 (Recovery dinner talk)

"This is what real family life looks like," Thabo shared, pointing to their messy whiteboard notes. *"Some days everything falls apart, and that's just part of the pattern too."*

The Truth About Numbers with Ava and Zach's 'Hospital Family'

Their Data told Honest Stories of a Tough Week:

    Monday: Missed dinner (emergency surgery)
    Tuesday: 10-minute connection only
    Wednesday: Family meal but everyone on devices
    Thursday: Quality time with one child, missed other
    Friday: Complete meltdown, but honest talk after
    Saturday: Recovery day, deep connections
    Sunday: Back to basics, simple presence

"These aren't failures to us," Ava insisted. *"They're data points helping us understand our family's true rhythms better so we can work on improving connection."*

The Recovery Protocol – The 'Hospital Healing' Zach and Ava Implemented at Home

After Missing Three Family Dinners:

- Acknowledgment: *"We're off track"*
- Assessment: Everyone shares impact
- Adjustment: Small changes identified
- Action: Simple next steps
- Acceptance: *"It's okay to be imperfect"*

"At times connection looks like sitting in silence after a huge fight," Ava noted. *"That counts too."*

The Technology Fails – When Thabo and Amara Faced Digital Family Overload

Weekend Screen Battle:

- Saturday morning: All devices dying
- Family tension rising
- Power bank politics
- Wi-Fi password standoff
- Unexpected outcome: Board games
- Connection found in disconnect

"Sometimes," Amara asserted, *"perceived system failure is really the system working."*

Growth Through Struggle - Keiko and Chen's Quake-proof Family Allowed for Tremors

Monthly Reality Check:

- Perfect days: 10%
- Good enough days: 55%
- Struggle days: 25%
- Crisis days: 10%

"Like seismic readings," Chen explained, *"the disruptions tell us as much as the calm periods."*

Key Takeaway 14: Strong partnerships make stable family systems - not through perfection, but resilient responses to imperfection. Strong families struggle but learn how to recover together.

CLOSING REFLECTION

As another messy dinner ends in their Osaka home, Hamish and Yuki watch their children clear the table - arguing, laughing, dropping things and making up. *"You know what real family engineering is?"* Yuki muses. *"Building kinship strong enough to hold all this beautiful chaos."*

Remember: The messy moments aren't system failures – they are where real family connection occurs. The most connected families aren't those with perfect systems, but those who keep trying, keep forgiving, keep starting over again.

In Chapter Fifteen, *Social Connection Architecture,* we'll explore how couples can maintain their partnership while building community connection. We will consider how resilient approaches to family life can strengthen our links beyond the home.

15

SOCIAL CONNECTION ARCHITECTURE

Social support, generosity to one another, and honest government are crucial for wellbeing

— WORLD HAPPINESS REPORT 2020

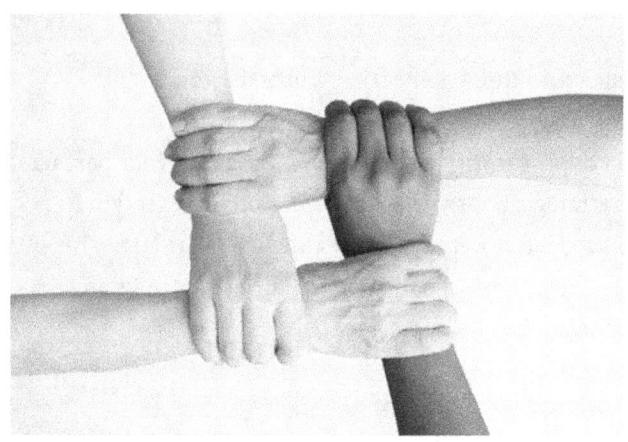

Real Life Scenario: The Community Bridge

"Sometimes the strongest connection happens through others," Thabo reflected, watching Amara organize their neighborhood's power-cut support group. Their home had become a hub where local families shared power banks, meals, and stories during electricity blackouts.

Socially-Minded High-Performance Couples Tend to Ask These Questions:

- How do we help other couples and causes while strengthening our own bond?
- What amount of social and community involvement is right for us and our children?

Overview

Strong relationship infrastructure includes robust external support systems. Social architecture isn't building a contacts list – it's designing community connections that reciprocally strengthen your partnership. This chapter focuses on how to engineer your social connections to support your relationship, while simultaneously fortifying your community wellbeing.

Your social connection engineering will assist you to:

- Form couple identity systems that strengthen your partnership
- Make strategic approaches to community integration
- Build supportive networks that enhance relationship resilience
- Clarify protocols for managing social relationships as a united team

COUPLE IDENTITY DEVELOPMENT

In the digital age, where relationships occur partly online, the architecture of social connection plays a pivotal role in shaping the quality and depth of our interactions. For high-performing, tech-savvy couples, the challenge lies not only in maintaining a vibrant connection with each other but also in fostering meaningful relationships beyond the confines of their partnership.

Couple Identity Development

This is rooted in the idea of 'we-ness,' encapsulating the shared identity and sense of unity within a partnership. This shared identity is not only a reflection of the individuals involved but also a dynamic entity that grows over time, shaped by shared experiences, values, and goals. Couple identity serves as the bedrock of a relationship, providing a sense of stability and cohesion amidst the ever-shifting landscape of modern life.

A key aspect of couple identity development is clarifying shared values and goals that guide your partnership. This dialogue lays the foundation for a couple vision, ensuring you are moving in the same direction and working towards mutually beneficial and agreed-upon outcomes. As you negotiate the difficulties of life together, your shared identity becomes a source of strength that enables you to approach challenges with a unified perspective and a sense of purpose.

Couple identity development is also forged through rituals and traditions that reinforce your connection. These rituals anchor your relationship, thickening your bond and creating continuity that transcends the day-to-day demands of work, family, and social obligations.

Reflection:

Take some time to reflect on the values, goals and experiences that define your relationship.

Discuss these with your partner and work together to write a one paragraph long couple identity statement that captures the essence of your partnership. Use this statement to guide your lives together, reviewing it often to keep it true to your ultimate stories, values and hopes.

COMMUNITY INTEGRATION STRATEGIES

Ironically, in our internet-linked world where technology facilitates global interactions – many people live in isolation. This makes integration into our communities more vital than ever to the health of relationships. For couples immersed in professional pursuits, community integration may seem secondary. However, it is through these local engagements that you can grow a sense of belonging and purpose – reaching beyond the confines of your personal bond.

Engaging with your community is to value local connectedness. Participation in events like festivals, farmers' markets, spiritual or cultural gatherings can lead to meaningful interactions with others. These kinds of activities help you build friendships that enlarge your social circles, increasing a sense of solidarity and purpose. For example, as a couple and family, we have found great support through our local school, sporting, church, work and cultural communities.

Volunteering is a key to local community involvement, by giving your time and skills to promote causes that matter to you while connecting with like-minded others. Whether in a local cleanup, mentoring youth, or supporting a food bank, volunteering together supports your community in tangible ways, reinforcing your bond while benefiting others.

Supporting local businesses and artisans also builds community integration. In markets often dominated by global enterprises, patronizing neighborhood shops and restaurants boosts the local economy and personal ties with those who live and work nearby. By getting to know the faces behind the products and services you enjoy, you build links via routine transactions.

Taking part in civic leadership and advocacy initiatives is another way to connect as a couple in the broader social landscape. Staying informed about issues and participating in local forums lets you show commitment to the welfare of your community. This supports positive change and connects you with those dedicated to improving the socio-cultural fabric of your area.

SUPPORT NETWORK BUILDING

For high-achieving couples, a network of reliable friends is a life support system of emotional care, practical help, and opportunities for personal growth. Building this support system starts with finding folks who enrich your life and offer diverse perspectives. These may include family members, lifelong friends, mentors, or colleagues – who share your values.

While technology can help, personalized communication is best. Taking time to meet in person, even for a brief coffee or shared meal, adds a depth to relationships that digital interactions cannot provide. These face-to-face encounters foster emotional intimacy and understanding, strengthening the bonds that form the backbone of your support network.

Beyond individual relationships - group interactions, social gatherings, community events, or professional meetups can expand your network and give you new perspectives. Such exchanges can bolster existing connections and help you forge new ones. Engaging with a diverse range of people will enrich your worldview, enabling you to draw on varied experiences and insights.

While building your support network, remember that reciprocity is key - relationships are a two-way street, needing mutual support and understanding. Being there for others in their times of need, offering your skills, resources or listening ear are all ways to deepen your connections, enhance the well-being of others, and grow social cohesion.

Research has shown that people with robust social support systems experience better health outcomes, greater resilience, and enhanced well-being. These benefits are especially pertinent for couples juggling multiple responsibilities, as strong support provides a cushion against stress and adversity, allowing you to thrive both individually and together.

Couple Identity in Community – Noticing Progress with Three of our Couples:

Remember how Thabo and Amara initially struggled with cultural integration? Their community role transformed as their couple identity journey strengthened over an 18-month period. *"We stopped trying to fit in,"* Amara reflected, *and started making space for people to belong."*

Neighborhood Involvement Journey

Stage	Challenge	Growth	Outcome
Initial	Cultural clash	Found allies	Bridge builders
Middle	Work-home balance	Shared struggles	Became mentors
Current	Family-community	Created spaces	Community anchors

Zach & Ava's social connection tracking also revealed surprising patterns as they discovered their emergency room connections rippled gently outward to become a real community web.

Professional	Personal	Unexpected Gain
Staff support	Babysitting swap	Marriage mentors
Parent groups	Date night coverage	Cultural bridges
Crisis teams	Holiday celebrations	Extended family

COUPLE IDENTITY IN COMMUNITY - NOTICING PROGRESS WITH THREE OF OUR COUPLES

"We thought we were just surviving shifts," Ava shared, *"but we were building our village."*

Hamish and Yuki's community integration, while tentative, yielded benefits beyond the costs, in a cross-cultural environment where their family needed more support.

The Cultural Bridge Builders

What Worked	What Didn't	What Surprised
Monthly potluck	Formal events	Random coffee meets
Kid playdates	Cultural classes	School gate chats
Festival help	Committee roles	Family crisis support

"What we hoped would help us feel accepted didn't work," Hamish commented, *"but little bits of regular connection around food and chatting made our family feel included after about one year here. What a relief for our family to feel settled, like we could really put our roots down."*

Action Steps:

1. Today

- Note one community connection
- Accept one social invitation
- Reach out to one supporter
- Swap one 'duty' for some fun

2. This Week

- Map your actual support network
- Identify gaps and strengths
- Make one small connection
- Honor boundaries that work

184 | SOCIAL CONNECTION ARCHITECTURE

3. This Month

- Review community involvement
- Adjust commitments to reality
- Strengthen key relationships
- Release obligations that drain

Success Metrics - Examples for You to Consider Tracking Monthly

Connection Type	Target	Acceptable Reality
Deep friendships	3-4	1-2 quality bonds
Community roles	1-2	1 meaningful position
Support circles	Various	Two reliable ones
Social events	Monthly	When energy permits

CLOSING REFLECTION

As evening settles over their Johannesburg suburb, Thabo & Amara watch their local community gather for an impromptu crisis preparedness meeting. What started as practical planning has evolved into something deeper.

"Look at us all," Thabo muses, *"different cultures, careers, beliefs - all connected by caring about each other's safety."* Amara nods, remembering how their professional expertise in IT and finance unexpectedly made them community anchors.

Key Takeaway 15: External relationships boost internal bonds, not by perfect social performance, but with genuine community connection that honors partnership and personal needs.

Remember: Just as power supply is vital yet varies, relationships grow by flexible connections to their communities. Your social architecture doesn't need to be perfect - just real. The most connected couples aren't those with the busiest social calendars, but those who've found their authentic place in their communities.

In Chapter Sixteen: *Advanced Connection Engineering,* we'll explore how couples take their relationship mastery to the next level. We'll see how the community wisdom we've gathered combines with our previous learning about crisis-proofing, career integration, and family systems, to create truly unshakeable partnerships.

16

ADVANCED CONNECTION ENGINEERING

Imagine you woke up tomorrow and your best hopes are fulfilled in the best possible ways. What are all the things you would notice, that would tell you that your preferred future is here?

— SUSANNE BURGSTALLER & CHRIS IVESON

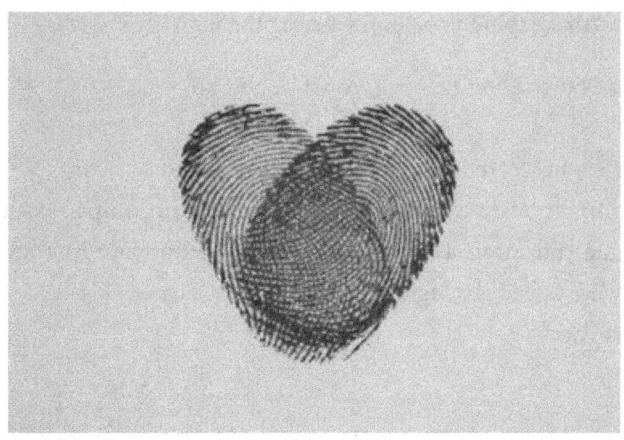

Real Life Scenario:

In Tokyo, Keiko and Chen began their careers and relationship with rigid engineering principles. *"Remember our first earthquake?"* Keiko laughs now. *"We tried to calculate everything. Now we feel the building's dance and just move with it."*

Their Journey Map Shows Real Transformation

Starting Point	Middle Ground	Current Reality
Fear tremors	Accept shaking	Flow with earth
Plan connection	Allow space	Trust rhythm
Fix all problems	Shift patterns	Grow naturally

Overview

Mastery in any engineering discipline requires advancing beyond basic principles to innovative applications. This chapter lifts your relationship engineering skills to expert level, helping you create cutting-edge connection strategies for the preferred future of your partnership.

Advanced engineering isn't about complexity, but sophisticated simplicity that earns compound interest over time. Mastering advanced techniques and innovation strategies will help you build connection architecture for future growth, keeping your bond strong through life's stages.

Through advanced engineering, you'll be able to:

- Hone sophisticated love habits that compound over time
- Develop innovative bonding systems for relationship growth
- Imagine your preferred future together to fulfil your best hopes
- Apply advanced strategies for continuous relationship progression

This chapter completes your transformation from relationship builder to relationship architect, equipping you with the highest level of connection engineering expertise.

High-Performing Couples Committed to Next-Level Relating Have Asked:

- How can we build on our strong base to go even further in deepening our connection?
- How might we support other couples who need mentoring or a bit of guidance at times?

NEXT-LEVEL INTIMACY TECHNIQUES

We all know innovation drives success in business, yet it's easy to overlook the equally valid need for ingenuity in personal relationships. This is where advanced connection engineering employs the strategic planning that fuels your work to exponentially increase couple intimacy while helping you mentor others who are seeking to renew their relationship.

Next-Level Intimacy Techniques

Within the dance of successful relationships, intimacy is often the focal point of attention and creativity. The key to deepening closeness is to grasp the many facets of connection and move from performance-based acts to engage all your senses. This grows emotional glue, more holistic engagement and an embodied experience of oneness deeper than just the physical.

Incorporating techniques from sex therapy such as sensate focus exercises can reduce anxiety by concentrating on somatic experiences and non-verbal communication. These exercises, developed by Dr. William Masters and Dr. Virginia Johnson, teach being present and attuned to your partner's bodily signals, for deeper emotional and physical connection. Focusing on each other's touch, scent and presence, can help deepen bonding on every level.

190 | ADVANCED CONNECTION ENGINEERING

Techniques like mindful breathing and visualization can be calming and create a safe space for vulnerability and openness. These practices nurture the emotional peace and presence that help both partners to explore their desires and boundaries with confidence.

Effective communication is the heart of any strong relationship, hence refining this skill will boost the quality of your intimacy. Practices like Nonviolent Communication (NVC) promote empathy and understanding, enabling couples to express their needs and desires without criticism. This strengthens the trust, emotional connection and security in the relationship.

Reflection Exercise:

Dedicate 15 minutes to reflect on your experiences and feelings regarding intimacy.

At what moments have you felt most connected to your partner and what contributed to that?

Note these and share them together, then adjust or explore new ways to nurture each other.

INNOVATION IN CONNECTION PRACTICES

While relentlessly pursuing career success, it's easy to overlook the need for innovation in personal relationships, but just as the tech world thrives on creativity, so can your relationship. Freshness in your relating comes via small, meaningful acts that infuse your partnership with new energy, like tweaking your morning **6MC, Midday Check-in** or evening exercise routine.

Creative collaboration, as applied in successful workplaces, also enriches couple connection. Working together on projects, whether home improvement, planning a trip, voluntary service or starting a small business, can foster a sense of teamwork and purpose.

Another innovative practice is using gamification in your relationship, such as friendly competitions that help you engage in novel ways. Whether a fitness challenge, a cooking contest, or reading marathon, these kinds of activities inject fun and excitement, humor and playfulness into your interactions, which relieve stress and create a lighter atmosphere.

Cultural exploration can also serve as a rich avenue for connection. Engaging with new cultures, whether via travel, cooking international cuisine, or attending festivals, can expand your horizons and deepen your understanding of others. Sharing these discoveries with friends and family can further strengthen your social network – the broader context for your partnership.

Further, the power of storytelling - sharing personal narratives and family histories can reveal hidden facets of your identity that enhance empathy. By weaving your stories together, you create a fund of shared experiences that enrich your bond. This practice of exchanging stories can remind you of your couple journey, highlighting how you have grown and changed.

IMAGINING YOUR PREFERRED FUTURE

Start by exploring your best hopes for your future together, through candid conversations about your aspirations and dreams. This dialogue is both an event and an ongoing imaginative conversation that adapts as circumstances change. By exploring your hopes, you can create a pathway that guides your decisions and reinforces your commitment to one another.

Action Steps:

Review the *10 Dimensions of Wellbeing* from your *Whole of System Assessment* and ask each other, *"What does our preferred future look like - to you?"* in a few of those key aspects.

192 | ADVANCED CONNECTION ENGINEERING

For example, maintaining financial wellbeing is a core component of couple relationships.

Money can be a major stressor for couples, and addressing financial concerns proactively can stop them from becoming a source of conflict. Short and simple talks about your money goals, budgets, spending, saving and investing, can help you agree on financial plans that meet short-term needs and long-range hopes, creating a sense of shared responsibility and security.

Investing in continuous learning and personal development will also help you forge the future you prefer in your relationship. Encourage each other to pursue new skills and opportunities that align with your individual and collective goals. This growth will enhance your fulfilment and enrich your partnership by bringing fresh perspectives and experiences into the mix.

Lastly, plan to regularly check the health of your relationship and address any concerns. By actively engaging in this process – 'little and often' - you demonstrate commitment to nurturing a relationship that is not only resilient but also deeply rewarding and models health to others.

ADVANCED CONNECTION ENGINEERING - CELEBRATING MASTERY WITH TWO OF OUR COUPLES

Beyond the Basics - Keiko and Chen Found New Depths in their Quake-Proof Love:

Early Years	Middle Stage	Advanced Level
Crisis response	Pattern recognition	Preventative design
Basic tools	Integrated systems	Innovative solutions
Surface fixes	Deep renovation	Continuous progression

"We thought we knew engineering," Chen smiled, reviewing their relationship blueprints. "Then life and 20 years of marriage taught us about quantum mechanics in love."

Where To From Here?

Keiko and Chen's earthquake engineering offers a final metaphor. *"Each tremor teaches us,"* Chen reflects, *"Not just about buildings, but about life's constant motion."* Their future aim is to:

- Trust more, control less
- Feel deeply, plan lightly
- Build wisdom, share freely
- Love fully, grow naturally

Keiko and Chen discovered intimacy at earthquake frequency. *"Like seismic waves,"* Keiko explained, *"the deepest connections happen below the surface - beyond where we can see."*

The Masters' Journey of Innovation in Connection for Zach and Ava

"We learned to read vital signs," Ava shared during their midnight rounds. *"Now we read whole of life signs - the subtle shifts that signal we have deeper connection needs."*

Zach and Ava's emergency medicine wisdom progressed into relationship mastery.

The Ripple Effect

Remember how Zach and Ava's hospital connection points spread through their community?

Legacy in Action

Personal Growth	Community Impact	Global Ripples
Better listening	Mentor new staff	Teaching model
Crisis strength	Support groups	Published study
Loving wisdom	Family networks	Training others

"Sometimes," Ava shared during handover, *"our smallest moments make the biggest changes."*

"In trauma medicine," Zach mused, *"there's a moment when everything stops - when even time holds its breath. We found that space in love too and want others to be able to learn it also."*

CLOSING REFLECTION

In their Tokyo apartment, as another small tremor ripples through the building, Keiko and Chen share a moment of profound understanding. Their advanced seismic monitors remain quiet - this shake is too subtle for instruments to detect. Yet they feel it together, their connection tuned to earth's gentlest whispers.

"This is what mastery means," Keiko muses. *"Not controlling these earthquakes, but dancing with them."* Chen nods, remembering how they once feared these tremors. Now each one deepens their trust in their relational foundations.

Key Takeaway 16: Intentional continuous improvement strengthens relationship resilience through natural growth and maturing rather than forced change.

Remember: Healthy connections are lovingly grown and nurtured to flourish and reproduce.

In our CONCLUSION, *Your Engineering Legacy*, we'll explore how these advanced practices can create lasting legacies of love. We'll see how the wisdom from each stage of *Couple Connection Mastery* can be shared, making ripples of renewal in families, communities, and generations.

Your 28-Day Transformation Roadmap – Completed. Well Done!

Week 1: Getting Started

- Day 1-3: Assessment ✅
- Day 4-7: Goal setting ✅
- Action focus: Morning rituals ✅

Week 2: Establishing Habits

- Day 8-14: Practice recording ✅
- Implementation focus: Daytime connection ✅
- Family rhythm integration ✅

Week 3: Optimizing Connection

- Day 15-21: System optimization ✅
- Strategic refinement: Evening habits ✅
- Family adaptation support ✅

Week 4: Consolidation and Celebration

- Day 22-28: Success amplification ✅
- Sustainable integration: Routine set ✅
- Longterm connection enhancement ✅

You Did It – Congratulations!

MAKE A DIFFERENCE WITH YOUR REVIEW - UNLOCK COUPLE CONNECTION FOR OTHERS

"A strong relationship isn't built in a day - it's built every day"

— UNKNOWN

Every relationship grows stronger with warm encouragement, and your words can make a real difference.

Would you help someone just like yourselves - an ambitious, analytically minded couple looking to reconnect but unsure where to start?

My mission is to make *Couple Connection Mastery* accessible to every couple seeking to strengthen their bond. But to reach more people, I need your help.

Most people choose books based on reviews. That means your review could be a key to helping more couples start on the path toward stronger trust, deeper intimacy and better communication. It takes one minute, but its impact could be life-changing.

Your review could help…

- …one more couple turn distance into closeness.
- …one more partnership engineer unbreakable love.
- …one more family create a healthier happier home.
- …one more dream of a thriving relationship come true.

To make a difference, simply scan the E-Book or Paper Back QR code below and leave a review

If you believe in the power of *Couple Connection,* you're my kind of person. Thank you from the bottom of my heart!

Daryl Parsons

CONCLUSION

17

YOUR ENGINEERING LEGACY

These trees which he plants, and under whose shade he shall never sit, he loves them for themselves, and for the sake of his children and his children's children, who are to sit beneath the shadow of their spreading boughs

— HYACINTHE LOYSON

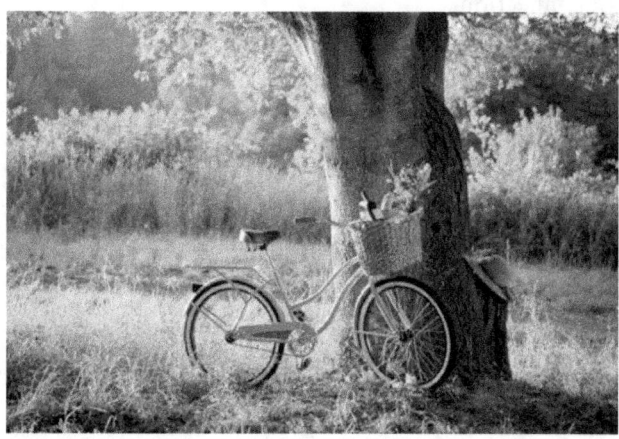

Overview

Every great engineering achievement leaves a lasting legacy, and your renewed relationship is no exception. This conclusion chapter helps you solidify your relationship engineering mastery while strengthening systems for continued growth and positive impact beyond your partnership.

Legacy building isn't just about maintaining what you've created, it's about self-growing systems that continue to bolster your connection through every life stage. By implementing continuous improvement protocols and future growth strategies, you ensure your relationship engineering skills keep advancing long after completing this initial renewal process.

Engineering your legacy will help you:

- Maintain sustainable systems for ongoing relationship growth
- Creatively use the BUILD framework for innovative connection
- Consider strategies for sharing your learning with others

This marks not an ending but a new step of your ongoing journey as a relationship engineer, equipped with tools and strategies to serve you for a lifetime of connection.

VALUING YOUR ENGINEERING LEGACY AS A TREASURE TO SHARE

As a couple, you represent countless others striving to translate high performance and strategic planning principles from their work into their relationships. As you solidify your own engineering legacy, let's review your progress thus far. The goal was improving your trust, communication and intimacy while creating a foundation as strong as the most resilient structures ever built.

Your Road to Relationship Renewal

We began with the big picture *'Whole of System Time Use and Life Quality Assessment.'* From that, the DECODE phase invited you to pause and reflect on the subtle drift that often creeps into relationships - what we term 'Partnership Drift.' Then you learned to recognize the signs of emotional disengagement and the logistics-only trap that reduce meaningful interaction to mundane exchanges. By understanding the science of connection and measuring the vitality of your relationship, you established baseline metrics for checking your progress.

Transitioning into the ENGINEER phase, you applied the Relationship BUILD framework, a structured yet flexible approach to reinvigorating your partnership. By recording your metrics and goals, understanding your partner's needs, and implementing strategic connection points, you worked to leverage strengths and deepen bonds. Finally, the FORTIFY phase equipped you with tools to crisis-proof your connection, integrate career and home life, and build a support network that enriches your relationship. This progression from recognition to active engagement and innovation exemplifies the transformative power of purposeful connection.

Throughout this pathway, you have shown commitment to growth and an unwavering belief in the potential of your partnership. You have enacted the core tenets of *Building a Life You Want: The Principles of Life Engineering*, applying its philosophy in your relationship. By cultivating love habits, nurturing meaningful connections, and fostering a growth mindset, you have crafted a legacy reaching beyond the edges of your partnership, influencing the lives of those around you.

In doing this, *you've not only engineered a stronger relationship but also developed a new way of doing partnership that honors your drive for excellence and desire for meaningful connection.* The systems and protocols you've built will keep supporting your relationship's growth while inspiring others to improve their relationships with similar precision and purpose.

MAINTAINING MOMENTUM

In your busy life, carving out time for your relationship has been hard. Yet, like any well-oiled machine, the key to maintaining momentum lies in consistent upkeep and mindful attention. The routines you've established through this process are now the pillars that support your relationship's ongoing growth. Keep weaving these small but significant practices into your daily life, ensuring they don't stay in this book, but become normalized parts of who you are.

Just as you would review a project roadmap at work, regularly revisiting these love habits can keep them relevant and effective. It is vital to keep evaluating what works and what doesn't, then adjusting as life inevitably changes. Regular check-ins are essential - not just with each other but also with yourself. These pauses for reflection offer insight into what's thriving and what needs nurturing, providing a clear view of your relationship's health.

As you move forward, the interplay of work, family, and personal wellbeing is so crucial. That's why I demonstrated it with the '*10 Dimensions of Wellbeing*' in my '*Whole of System*' approach to life and health. This is more than sharing hours between work and home - it's about integrating all aspects of life in ways that feel satisfying and sustainable. Holistic wellbeing is clearly a societal task as well as an individual and couple one, hence it requires teamwork.

Reflection Questions:

Looking back on the 'Whole of System Overview' you did at the start – how much has your Holistic Wellbeing / Quality of Life Score improved, at the end of our 28-Day Roadmap?

Reviewing your 28-Day Roadmap in Chapter 6 – how much have your metric scores improved?

The demands of your career are significant, and the responsibilities of family can feel weighty. Viewing these not as competing forces but as complementary parts of a fulfilling life can change the narrative. *This perspective shift allows you to see how your professional skills - planning, prioritizing, and communicating - can enrich all of your life.* Using these at home can create harmony where all areas of your life enhance each other. For instance, just as you schedule important work meetings, planning time for your partner ensures connection stays top priority.

Incorporating technology thoughtfully into your relationship can help you maintain momentum. As someone attuned to the latest innovations, you understand the power of technology to keep people connected across distances. Leverage this to your advantage, while setting boundaries to stop it distracting you, designating tech-free times and zones to focus solely on each other.

Physical and mental wellness are equally vital in sustaining the energy needed to keep your relationship thriving. Regular exercise, mindful practices, and healthy nutrition are not just personal goals but shared pursuits that can strengthen your bond. Engaging in activities that promote physical and mental health can boost connection. Reflective practices like meditation or journaling can provide clarity and reduce stress. By prioritizing wellness together, you build foundations that support individual and collective well-being.

Social interactions and community involvement help sustain your relationship momentum. Engaging with friends, family, and community members expands your support network, offering diverse perspectives and shared experiences that enrich your life together. These connections remind you of the broader context in which your relationship exists, just as participating in cultural and spiritual activities deepens your connection in ways that resonate profoundly.

CREATING LASTING IMPACT

Creating a lasting impact within your relationship is akin to planting seeds that will grow into a flourishing garden, that nurtures not just you and your partner but also the world around you.

As you cultivate a life worth living, how may your relationship extend its influence beyond the immediate confines of your personal space to make the world a better place?

Reflect on the values and practices that have guided you through this renewal. These habits can inspire change and positivity in your broader community. When you and your partner model healthy communication, mutual respect, and empathy, you set a powerful example for others.

This influence is not limited to those in your immediate circle but can ripple outward, touching the lives of friends, colleagues, and even strangers who observe your interactions. I have seen the power of this. Your relationship becomes a beacon of what is possible when two individuals commit to growth and learning, exciting others to seek similar progress in their own lives.

The concept of legacy is often associated with tangible achievements, yet the most profound legacies are those that shape the attitudes and behaviors of others, leaving a mark on the collective consciousness.

Review the moments when you and your partner have overcome challenges, celebrated victories, or simply supported each other through life's ebbs and flows.

These experiences, though personal, have the potential to enrich the lives of those around you. By sharing your triumphs and trials, you offer valuable insights and encouragement to others walking similar paths. Whether through casual conversations, social media, or more formal avenues like workshops or community groups, your story can be a source of inspiration and learning. This is not about boasting or seeking validation, but offering hope and showing that meaningful, loving relationships are attainable despite life's demands. *Many need to see this.*

At the heart of creating a lasting impact is recognizing no relationship exists in isolation. The choices you make and the values you uphold contribute to a collective narrative influencing broader society. Relating grounded in love, respect, and growth not only enriches your own lives but also contributes to a more compassionate and connected world. As you continue to build on the foundation you have established, remember that the true measure of your relationship's success lies not just in personal fulfilment but in the positive change it inspires in others.

As you continue this journey, remember the actionable strategies and practices that we have shared. Your daily connection rituals serve as anchors, grounding your relationship amidst the ever-changing tides of life. Vulnerability, once perceived as a weakness, becomes a powerful tool for deepening intimacy and fostering trust. Use change as a chance to grow and keep open to new experiences that enrich your connection. By doing so, you create a dynamic partnership capable of weathering the storms of life and emerging stronger and more resilient.

Further Application

I encourage you to view this book not as a one-time read, but as a guide to revisit and reference as your relationship develops. The exercises and habits provided are designed to be adapted to your unique circumstances, so keep using the exercises that helped you. Set goals for the next stage of your relationship journey, whether it's establishing a new daily ritual, engaging in open dialogue, or exploring new avenues for connection, the key is action. *Love is a verb.*

WHAT YOU DO LOCALLY CAN HELP COUPLE CONNECTION IMPROVE GLOBALLY

Reflecting on my journey and the insights gained through authoring this book, I am filled with joy and gratitude for the opportunity to share this knowledge with you. As a former carpenter turned counsellor and educator, I have witnessed firsthand the enduring impact and legacy of these principles in my own life and the lives of countless couples I have worked with.

The journey from constructing physical structures to building the emotional architecture of relationships has taught me that the base of any strong partnership lies in the willingness to grow, learn, and invest in each other. I hope that the strategies and insights shared in this book serve as a guiding light, illuminating your path to a deeper and more meaningful connection.

If you have found applying this book helpful in any way, please leave a Review using the QR Code provided and recommend it to those who want to reconnect their couple relationship. Thanks.

As you start the next chapter of your relationship, I invite you to connect with me by email. I would appreciate hearing what has helped you most to grow and what your couple connection is like now, compared with before you read and applied this book. Email on: info@darylparsons.com

Finally, I extend my heartfelt gratitude for your commitment to enhancing your relationship. Your dedication to love and connection is a testament to the resilience of the human spirit. As you move forward, carry with you the optimism and confidence that comes from knowing you possess the tools and supports to engineer an unbreakable bond.

In the *Appendices* that follow, you will find valuable resources to help your ongoing journey. Most importantly, I have provided a collection of the *'Connection Assessment Tools'* we used to evaluate and track your relationship's progress. You can copy and use these to record your metrics for further advancement. Details of the Couples in our Case Studies are in Appendix B.

Remember:

Your journey continues.
Your love matters supremely.
Your connection creates legacy.
Build strongly.
Love deeply.
Trust wisely.

May your love story be one of resilience, joy, and endless growth.

Together, let us create a world where thriving relationships help build a more compassionate, connected, courageous and creative society for the benefit and wellbeing of all.

With my gratitude and optimism, Daryl Parsons. Christchurch, New Zealand. March 2025

APPENDICES

RESOURCES FOR YOUR NEXT STEPS

Here I provide copies of the Connection Assessment Tools we used throughout the book to help you evaluate and track your relationship's progress over the months and years ahead..

Appendix A – Connection Assessment Tools:

The following *Connection Assessment Tools* are those we completed in our *Introduction*.

Assess Couple Connection within Your Whole of System - Time Use and Life Quality

Wellbeing Aspect	Human Behaviours	Daily Being-Doing	Daily	Weekly	Quality
Physical-Bodily	Bodily health actions	Sleep; food prep; eat-drink; wash; toilet;			
Mental-Emotional	Thinking-feeling-choosing				
Work-Study-Career	Vocation-calling-purpose				
Familial-Generational	Family-relatives-support				
Relational-Sexual	Couplehood-singlehood				
Home-Assets-Financial	Property-bills-investments				
Fun-Rest-Recreational	Exercise-hobbies-sports				
Spiritual-Cultural	Stories-values-practices				
Social-Friends	Friend-community activities				
Natural-Ecological	Plants-animals-land-care				
Overall Quality of Life in 10 Dimensions with Total Time Use Daily / Weekly:			= 24 Hrs	=168 Hrs	

PARSONS INDIVIDUAL AND SOCIETAL HOLISTIC WELLBEING SCALE

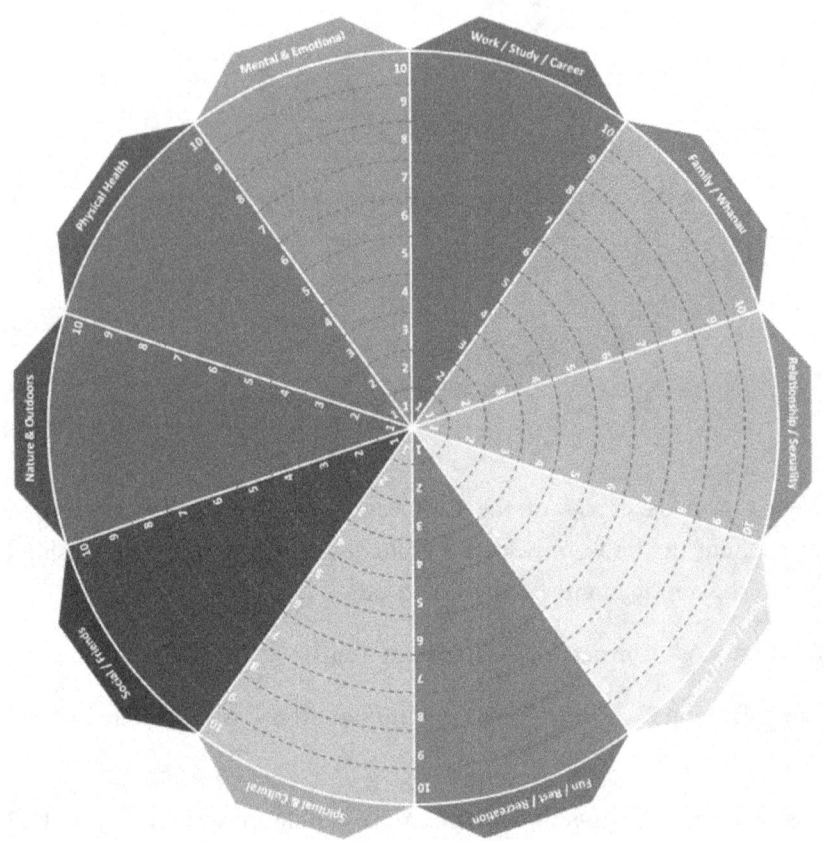

Appreciating and Strengthening Your Holistic Wellbeing – Towards Societal Wellbeing:

- How would you rate your Wellbeing in each related area, from 1 = Low, to 10 = High?
- Mark your scores on the Scale and join them up. What is your Wellbeing % Score?.....
- Appreciate what you have achieved, with your support people. Well done, great work!
- Next, what area – if strengthened, would help your life the most? ....
- Brainstorm, how might you do this? ....
- Support – who could help you? .... And who could you help? ....
- When will you achieve this by? .... Who will notice? ....
- Keep doing what works ☑ Check your progress often and update your support people

The following *Connection Assessment Tools* are those we used in Chapter Three and Eight.

RELATIONSHIP VITALITY DASHBOARD FOR COUPLE CONNECTION MASTERY

Having assessed your relationship vitality, let's bring your top seven metrics together in one place where you can see them in a one-stop-shop *Relationship Dashboard.* This Dashboard helps you view the key parts of your connection, to appreciate, assess and improve them.

The Text Connection Audit (15 minutes)

Text Topic	Contents of Our Last 20 Couple Text Messages	Stats	
Logistics	How many were purely logistical?	=	%
Emotional	How many contained emotional content?	=	%
Appreciation	How many expressed appreciation or affection?	=	%
Shared dreams	How many were about shared dreams or future plans?	=	%

212 | APPENDICES

Your 6-Minute Connect Trial - Record Your Notes Here:

Components to Practice	Quality and Impact	Relationship Satisfaction
First 2 Minutes: Present Moment	E.g Ok. Good. Helped	Low. Ok. Good. High. Great
Make eye contact over cuppa		
Share a full embrace		
Focus together - phones away		
2 Minutes: Emotional Check-In		
Share one hope for the day		
Express a concern or vulnerability		
Offer supporting acknowledgment		
2 Minutes: Thankful & Intention		
Express gratitude for recent thing		
Set connection intention for today		
Meaningful physical contact		
Overall – How was Your '6-Minute	Morning Connect?'	You Feel?

Connection Baseline – Taken Before Your 3-Day Challenge:

Connection Method	Baseline Metrics on Top Five Couple Connection Methods	Stats
Non-logistic chats	How many of your conversations were non-logistical per day?	
Focused attention	How many minutes of focused attention (no-devices) per day?	
Emotional sharing	How often did we share emotional thoughts / feelings daily?	
Meaningful touch	How many times of affectionate physical contact per day?	
Shared playfulness	How many moments of mutual laughter or play per day?	

Utilizing BCPs - Record of Trial Week for Connection and Learning:

Daily Number of Successful BCPs	Average Quality of Each BCP Connection	Impact on Emotional State of Both Partners	Effect on Relationship Satisfaction Reported
Monday =			
Tuesday =			
Wednesday =			
Thursday =			
Friday =			
Saturday =			
Sunday =			
Average = /Day	Quality =		

APPENDICES | 213

Your Midday Check-In Example (Adapted 6MC). Record Your Trial Notes Here:

TWO SHORT CONNECTION STEPS	Quality and Impact	Relationship Satisfaction
Thankful Moment & Update	*E.g Ok. Good. Helped*	*E.g Ok. Good. High. Great*
Express gratitude for recent action		
Ask / say how morning tasks went		
Emotional Validate & Check-In		
Validate one feeling shared above		
Offer support and hope to connect		
Overall: How was Your 'Midday	**Connect?'**	**You Feel?**

Key Connection Indicators - KCIs - Record Your Metrics & Experiences Here:

THREE TYPES OF CONNECTION	Quantity and Quality	Relationship Satisfaction
Physical Connection Metrics	*E.g 1-2. Ok. Good. Helped*	*Low. Good. High. Great*
Daily affectionate touches		
Non-sexual physical affection		
Sleep proximity patterns		
Sexually intimate moments		
Emotional Connection Metrics		
Deep conversations initiated		
Vulnerable shares exchanged		
Supportive moments offered		
Joint parenting wins		
Mental Connection Metrics		
Shared decisions made		
Problems solved together		
Future plans discussed		
Parenting strategies aligned		
Overall: How is Your Three-Fold	**Connection?**	**You Feel?**

Scaling Trust, Intimacy and Communication in Light of Your Metrics Above

Review your recorded Metrics above, then Rate with your partner the resulting quality of these three connection ingredients on our: **Trust, Intimacy and Communication Scale (TICS).** Note: it is normal for partners to give different ratings on these connection vital signs - for discussion.

214 | APPENDICES

Trust Scale: 0 _____ 10 (10 = Best)

Intimacy Scale: 0 _____ 10

Communication Scale: 0 _____ 10

Combine your Metrics, Connection KCIs and TIC Scale to Rate Your Resulting

RELATIONSHIP VITALITY SCALE: 0 _____ 10 (10 = Best)

This is Your 28-Day Roadmap Chart for Recording Your Top Six Metrics On (from Chapter Six)

Recording Your Couple Connection Quality Across Your 28-Day Roadmap

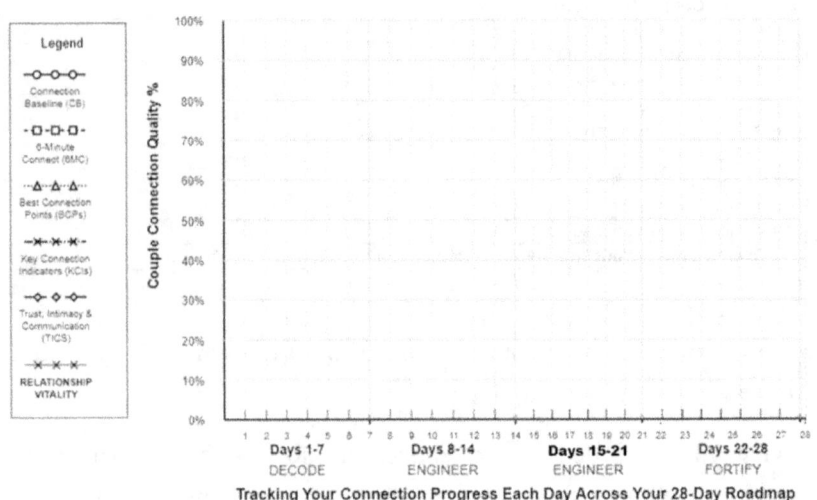

Tracking Your Connection Progress Each Day Across Your 28-Day Roadmap

For a printable copy of the Connection Assessment Tools in this book, scan this QR Code.

APPENDICES | 215

Appendix B – Our Case Study Couples' Locations and Professions

CHAPTER	NAMES	LOCATION	PROFESSIONS
Introduction - The Intimacy Achievement Paradox	Michael & Sarah	Christchurch, New Zealand	Managing Partner & CEO Tech
1 The Partnership Drift	Michael & Sarah	Christchurch, New Zealand	Managing Partner & CEO Tech
2 Time Starved Love	Jamie & Alex	Sydney, Australia	Surgeon Managing Director
3 The Science of Connection	Richard & Lisa	London, England	Conveyancing Lawyer Electrical Engineer
4 Engineering Love	Marcus & Maya	Boston, New England, USA	IT Analyst & CTO
5 The Relationship BUILD Framework	Elena & Wei	Kuala Lumpur, Malaysia	School Psychologist & Water Engineer
6 BASE – Foundation Setting	Thabo & Amara	Johannesburg, South Africa & Nigeria	IT Tech & CFO
7 UNDERSTAND – Connection Mapping	Yuki & Hamish	Osaka, Japan & Scotland	Textile Engineer Aerospace Engineer
8 IMPLEMENT – Strategic Connection Points	Omar & Freda	Zurich, (Türkiye) Switzerland	Landscape Architect Lecturer & Financier
9 LEVERAGE – System Optimization	Zach & Ava	Santiago, Chile	SMO Senior Doctor & Paediatric Specialist
10 DEEPEN – Architecture Strengthening	Keiko & Chen	Tokyo, Japan	Both Seismic Building Engineers
11 Crisis-Proofing Your Connection	James & Maria	Manila, Philippines	Both Meteorologists
12 Long-Distance Engineering	Moana & Kalani	Auckland, NZ & Oahu, Hawaii	Veterinary Science & Marine Biologist
13 Career-Connection Integration	Zach & Ava	Santiago, Chile	SMO Senior Doctor & Paediatric Specialist
14 Family System Integration	Yuki & Hamish	Osaka, Japan & Scotland	Textile Engineer & Aerospace Engineer
15 Social Connection Architecture	Thabo & Amara	Johannesburg, South Africa & Nigeria	IT Tech & CFO
16 Advanced Connection Engineering	Keiko & Chen	Tokyo Japan	Seismic Building Engineers

REFERENCES

Abundancetherapycenter.com. (n.d.). Navigating the impact of technology on relationships. https://www.abundancetherapycenter.com/blog/communication-and-the-impact-of-technology-on-relationships

Achiaa, F. (n.d.). Building an intentional legacy: Strategies and lasting impact for individuals and families. Medium. https://medium.com/@faithachiaa/building-an-intentional-legacy-strategies-and-lasting-impact-for-individuals-and-families-ec670a21ecf1

Amichai-Hamburger, Y., (2020). Daily technology interruptions and emotional and & Etgar, S relational well-being. Psychology & Health. https://pmc.ncbi.nlm.nih.gov/articles/PMC7430699/

Asaporg.com. (n.d.). How to set and maintain professional boundaries. https://www.asaporg.com/communication/how-to-set-and-maintain-professional-boundaries

Ascensioncounseling.com. (n.d.). Nurturing love: Daily steps with the Gottman method. https://ascensioncounseling.com/nurturing-love-daily-steps-with-the-gottman-method

Ascensioncounseling.com. (n.d.). Parenting partnership: Gottman method for couples. https://ascensioncounseling.com/parenting-partnership-gottman-method-for-couples

Bayareacbtcenter.com. (n.d.). Top sex therapy techniques to enhance intimacy. https://bayareacbtcenter.com/sex-therapy-techniques/

Botanicaweddings.com. (n.d.). 10 ways to futureproof your marriage. https://www.botanicaweddings.com/blog/10-ways-to-futureproof-your-marriage

Bruni, F. (2015, September 6). The myth of quality time. The New York Times. https://www.nytimes.com/2015/09/06/opinion/sunday/frank-bruni-the-myth-of-quality-time.html

Calmerry.com. (n.d.). Relationship crises: How to identify & deal with them. https://calmerry.com/blog/relationships/strategies-for-dealing-with-relationship-crises/

Campbell, K., & (2007). Couple rituals can strengthen the relationship. Ponzetti, J. J. Psychology Today. https://www.psychologytoday.com/us/blog/finding-love-the-scientific-take/202408/couple-rituals-can-strengthen-the-relationship

Catalystcenterllc.com. (n.d.). Strengthening relationships through the Gottman method. https://catalystcenterllc.com/strengthening-relationships-through-the-gottman-method/

Chadleyzobolastherapy.com. (n.d.). Managing stress as a couple: Strategies for balancing personal and relationship wellbeing. https://www.chadleyzobolastherapy.com/blog/managing-stress-as-a-couple-strategies-for-balancing-personal-and-relationship-wellbeing

Cliniclegal.org. (n.d.). 12 ways to promote integration in your community. https://www.clin

iclegal.org/resources/immigrant-integration/12-ways-promote-integration-your-community

Colorado State University. (n.d.). 10 ways to connect with your partner daily. https://source.colostate.edu/10-ways-connect-partner-daily/

Decideyourlegacy.com. (n.d.). 25 tips for strengthening relationships. https://decideyourlegacy.com/the-ultimate-guide-to-building-relationships/

Drjaci.com. (n.d.). Emotional bandwidth: A complete guide. https://drjaci.com/emotional-bandwidth/

Duke Human Resources. (n.d.). Balancing work & family. https://hr.duke.edu/wellness/mental-health-stress/success-over-stress/balancing-work-family/

Envisiontherapydfw.com. (n.d.). Work-life integration: Strategies for couples to thrive together. https://envisiontherapydfw.com/work-life-integration-strategies-for-couples-to-thrive-together/

Focus on the Family. (n.d.). Reconnect through meaningful conversation. https://www.focusonthefamily.com/marriage/reconnect-through-meaningful-conversation/

Fortune. (n.d.). 7 patterns a couples therapist found in lasting relationships. https://fortune.com/well/article/patterns-of-long-lasting-marriages/

Freedmarcroft.com. (n.d.). Top 10 ways to improve communication in your marriage. https://freedmarcroft.com/10-ways-to-improve-communication-in-your-marriage-and-strengthen-your-relationship/

Gapyearfamily.com. (n.d.). The nine qualities of highly successful families. https://www.gapyearfamily.com/the-nine-qualities-of-highly-successful-families/

Gottman, J. (n.d.). Healthy relationships in practice. Gottman Institute. https://www.gottman.com/blog/healthy-relationships-in-practice/

Gottman, J. (n.d.). Manage conflict: Identifying your triggers. Gottman Institute. https://www.gottman.com/blog/manage-conflict-triggers/

Gottman Institute. (n.d.). About the Gottman method. https://www.gottman.com/about/the-gottman-method/

Gottman Institute. (n.d.). Gottman relationship checkup - professionals. https://www.gottman.com/professionals/gottman-relationship-checkup/

Greenspacehealth.com. (n.d.). Relationship satisfaction assessment | RAS. https://greenspacehealth.com/en-us/relationship-satisfaction-ras/

Harvard Business (2023, Nov.).How creative collaboration can strengthen Review.relationships. https://hbr.org/2023/11/research-how-creative-collaboration-can-strengthen-relationships

Hedger, S. (n.d.). Performance coaching for couples. https://www.stephenhedger.com/performance-coaching-for-couples/

Holdinghopemft.com. (n.d.). Goal setting in relationships: A therapist's guide for couples. https://holdinghopemft.com/the-power-of-goal-setting-in-relationships-a-step-by-step-guide-for-couples/

Hprc-online.org. (n.d.). Optimize your "relationship" performance. https://www.hprc-online.org/total-force-fitness/gotmysix/resources/optimize-your-relationship-perfor mance

Huffpost.com. (n.d.). 12 healthy habits of couples who are in it for the long haul. https:// www.huffpost.com/entry/healthy-relationship-habits_l_5c64b8c7e4b0233af9713b31

Kansas University. (n.d.). Developing baseline measures of behavior. Community Tool Box http://ctb.ku.edu/en/table-of-contents/assessment/assessing-community-needs-and-resources/developing-baseline-measures/main

Kolb, D. A. (n.d.). Experiential learning cycle. Skills for Learning, Leeds Beckett University. http://skillsforlearning.leedsbeckett.ac.uk/preview/content/models/02.shtml

Marriage.com. (n.d.). 10 techniques for couples to align relationships and time. https:// www.marriage.com/advice/relationship/time-management-techniques-for-couples/

Marriage.com. (n.d.). 13 techniques to have productive relationship check-ins. https://www. marriage.com/advice/therapy/relationship-check-ins/

Marriage.com. (n.d.). 15 relationship rituals every couple should follow. https://www. marriage.com/advice/relationship/daily-relationship-rituals-for-couples-to-follow/

Marriagefamilyservices.com. (n.d.). Cultivating emotional intimacy in long-distance relationships. https://www.marriagefamilyservices.com/post/cultivating-emotional-intamacy-in-long-distance-relationships/

McKinsey & Company. (n.d.). How the best CEOs build lasting stakeholder relationships. https://www.mckinsey.com/capabilities/strategy-and-corporate-finance/our-insights/how-the-best-ceos-build-lasting-stakeholder-relationships

Modern Husbands. (n.d.). 31 simple time management hacks for married couples. https:// www.modernhusbands.com/post/31-simple-time-management-hacks-for-married-couples

Noldus.com. (n.d.). Understanding the micro-dynamics of couples' interactions. https:// www.noldus.com/blog/understanding-micro-dynamics-couples-interactions

NPR. (2022, March 14). Time management tips for busy working parents: Life kit. https:// www.npr.org/2022/03/14/1086480869/parents-are-exhausted-these-strategies-can-help-you-build-support-and-win-back-time

Paired.com. (n.d.). 24 apps for long-distance couples to stay connected. https://www.paired.com/articles/best-apps-for-long-distance-couples

Parivedasolutions.com. (n.d.). The giver framework: A strategy to build better relationships and organizations. https://parivedasolutions.com/perspectives/the-giver-framework-a-strategy-to-build-better-relationships-organizations/

Penn Today. (n.d.). 5 science-based tips for building love that lasts. https://penntoday.upenn.edu/news/five-science-based-tips-to-build-lasting-love

Petersorgenfrei.com. (n.d.). Balancing relationships and business growth: A guide to success. https://www.petersorgenfrei.com/post/balancing-relationships-and-business-growth-a-guide-to-success

Psychology Today. (n.d.). 5 essential traits of lasting relationships. https://www.psychologytoday.com/us/blog/communication-success/202110/5-essential-traits-lasting-relationships

220 | REFERENCES

Psychology Today. (n.d.). Setting SMART goals in your relationship. https://www.psychologytoday.com/us/blog/finding-love-the-scientific-take/202406/setting-smart-goals-in-your-relationship

Psychology Today. (n.d.). The psychology of strategic relationships. https://www.psychologytoday.com/us/blog/leadership-diversity-and-wellness/202412/the-psychology-of-strategic-relationships

Punde, A. (n.d.). Building a life you want: The principles of life engineering. LinkedIn. https://www.linkedin.com/pulse/building-life-you-want-principles-engineering-ashok-punde-9ll1f

Quickinsight.co. (n.d.).Balancing career ambitions with personal relationships. https://www.quickinsight.co/blog/balancing-career-ambitions-with-personal-relationships

Rdiconnect.com. (n.d.). Communicating effectively with extended family. https://www.rdiconnect.com/communicating-effectively-with-extended-family/

Regain.us. (n.d.). Telltale signs of emotional distance in relationships and how to bridge the gap. https://www.regain.us/advice/general/telltale-signs-of-emotional-distance-in-relationships-and-how-to-bridge-the-gap/

Re-thinkingthefuture.com. (n.d.). The role of architecture in promoting social interaction and community engagement. https://www.re-thinkingthefuture.com/architectural-community/a10744-the-role-of-architecture-in-promoting-social-interaction-and-community-engagement/

Sanberg, J. G., Novak, J. R., (2016). *Does couples' communication predict marital Harper, J. M., Holt-Lunstad, J., satisfaction, or does marital satisfaction predict & Brandon, T., communication?* Journal of Marital and Family Therapy, 42(3), 441-453. https://pmc.ncbi.nlm.nih.gov/articles/PMC4852543/

Silk, D., (2012) *Keep Your Love On: Connection, Communication and Boundaries.* Loving On Purpose, (p.51).

Smashing Magazine. (2011, May). Relationship engineering: Designing the happily ever after. https://www.smashingmagazine.com/2011/05/relationship-engineering-designing-the-happily-ever-after/

Southjerseycopingclinic.com. (n.d.). How to set goals and measure progress in couple's therapy. https://southjerseycopingclinic.com/how-to-set-goals-and-measure-progress-in-couples-therapy/

The 8080 Marriage. (n.d.). Shifting from logistics mode to intimacy mode in marriage. https://www.8080marriage.com/blog/Shifting-From-Logistics-Mode-to-Intimacy-Mode-in-Marriage

The Marriage Restoration (n.d.). Why presenting a united front with your husband or wife Project. is so important for a healthy relationship. https://themarriagerestorationproject.com/why-presenting-a-united-front-with-your-husband-or-wife-is-so-important-for-a-healthy-relationship/

The Sales Blog. (n.d.). Unscalable: How to build relationships at scale. https://www.thesalesblog.com/blog/unscalable-how-to-build-relationships-at-scale

Thriva.co. (n.d.). Implementation intentions: The science of 'if-then' planning. https://thriva.co/hub/behaviour-change/implementation-intentions

Tozer, D. (n.d.). 28 days get back to love intensive program. https://www.deetozer.com/28-days-get-back-to-love-intensive-program/

Travers, M. (2024, July 20). 3 'micro-moments' that create lasting relationships - by a psychologist. Forbes. https://www.forbes.com/sites/traversmark/2024/07/20/3-micro-moments-that-create-lasting-relationships-by-a-psychologist/

University at Buffalo (n.d.). Developing your support system. School of Social Work. https://socialwork.buffalo.edu/resources/self-care-starter-kit/additional-self-care-resources/developing-your-support-system.html

Vocal.media. (n.d.). How do you build emotional intimacy when you are going through a rough time. https://vocal.media/marriage/how-do-you-build-emotional-intimacy-when-you-are-going-through-a-rough-time-s553a0ace

Walko, E. (n.d.). Measuring "we-ness" in couple relationships: A social identity perspective. Journal of Marital and Family Therapy. https://pmc.ncbi.nlm.nih.gov/articles/PMC10946554/

Wired. (n.d.). How to use technology to fuel long-distance love. https://www.wired.com/story/how-to-use-technology-long-distance-relationships/

Zion & Zion. (n.d.). The impact of relationship building: A framework. https://www.zionandzion.com/the-impact-of-relationship-building-a-framework/

Zhong, J., & Baer, R., (2020). *Rituals and nuptials: The emotional and relational consequences of relationship rituals*. Journal of Consumer Research. https://www.journals.uchicago.edu/doi/abs/10.1086/702761

ALSO WRITTEN BY DARYL PARSONS

TO BUY THE KINDLE VERSION ON AMAZON.COM
CLICK THE QR CODE

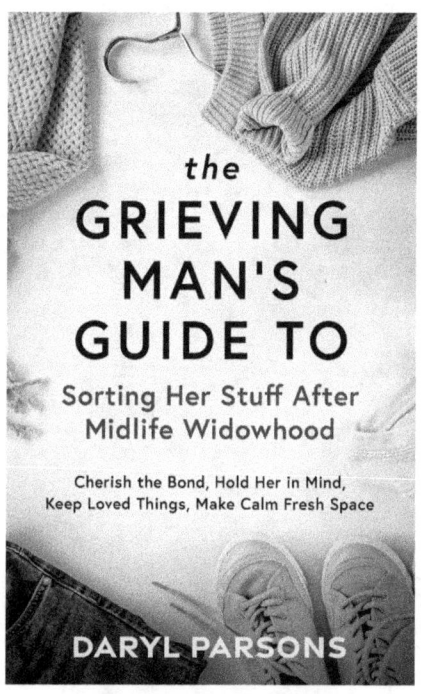

www.ingramcontent.com/pod-product-compliance
Lightning Source LLC
Chambersburg PA
CBHW050339010526
44119CB00049B/615